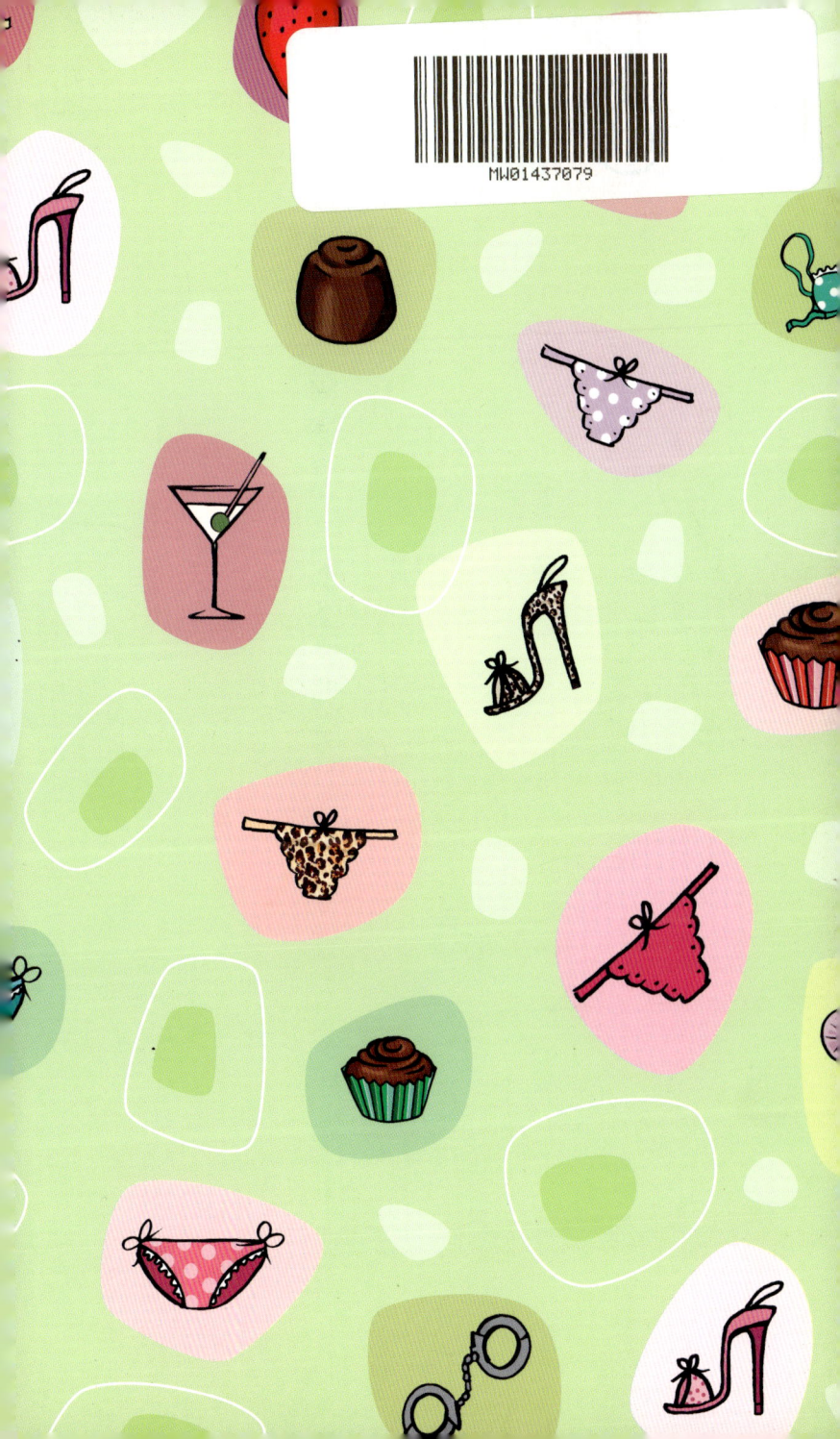

CLEO
Editor-In-Chief   Mia Freedman

ACP Books
Editorial Director   Susan Tomnay
Sales Director   Brian Cearnes
Production Manager   Carol Currie

Chief Executive Officer   John Alexander
Group Publisher   Pat Ingram
Publisher   Sue Wannan

Author   Charlotte Sherston

Editor   Deborah Bibby
Copy Editor   Jolanda Waskito
Designer   Timothy Clift - Swell Graphic Design (NSW)
Illustrator   Megan Hess - www.meganhess.com

Printed by Paramount Printing, Hong Kong.

Published by ACP Magazines Ltd, 54 Park Street, Sydney;
GPO Box 4088, Sydney, NSW 2001. Ph: (02) 9282 8618 Fax: (02) 9267 9438

www.acpbooks.com.au

To order books phone 136 116

AUSTRALIA: Distributed by Network Services, GPO Box 4088, Sydney, NSW 2001
Ph: (02) 9282 8777 Fax: (02) 9264 3278

NEW ZEALAND: Distributed by Southern Publishers Group
44 New North Road, Eden Terrace, Auckland. Ph: (649) 309 6930 Fax: (649) 309 6170
Email: hub@spg.co.nz

RIGHTS ENQUIRIES: Laura Bamford, Director ACP Books
Email: lbamford@acplon.co.uk Ph: +44 (207) 8126526

Sherston, Charlotte.

I'll have what she's having.

ISBN 1 86396 504 1.

1. Sex instruction for women. I. Title.

306.7

©ACP Magazines Ltd 2005
ABN 18 053 273 546

This publication is copyright. No part of it may be reproduced or transmitted in any
form without the written permission of the publishers.

I'll Have What She's Having

CHARLOTTE SHERSTON

Contents

CHAPTER 1 8
The Sound of One Hand
The DIY guide to masturbation

CHAPTER 2 22
How To Get Your Engine Started
Foreplay

CHAPTER 3 40
The Main Event
Sex - a beginner's guide

CHAPTER 4 60
I'll Have What She's Having
Orgasms

CHAPTER 5 80
Game Boy Advanced
Ways to drive him wild

CHAPTER 6 100
Light Her Fire
Ways to drive her wild

CHAPTER 7 120
Batteries Not Included
Toys, services and other stuff

CHAPTER 8 138
Protect Your Assets
Safe sex

CHAPTER 9 160
Batting For The Other Team
Gay, Lesbian, Bi-Sexual... are you or aren't you?

CHAPTER 10 176
When Good Sex Goes Bad
What can go wrong?
The do's and don'ts of sex

BIBLIOGRAPHY 198

CONTACT LIST 199

Introduction

IT IS A TRUTH UNIVERSALLY ACKNOWLEDGED THAT EVERYONE IS HAVING BETTER SEX THAN YOU ARE.

They are all swinging from the chandeliers in matching lingerie and climaxing in unison. Whilst you are a bit bored in your Bonds knickers that are no longer white. Or wondering why you are back shagging your ex-boyfriend who wasn't even that great first time round. Or having nice, cosy, predictable sex because you are too tired and have run out of tricks.

I have to admit, I always thought of myself as a pretty good shag. I thought I knew how to make a man (and myself on occasion) pretty damn happy. I thought I knew everything about sex from A-Z. I soon discovered, alphabetically speaking, I'd only really got as far as K. My own sex life began to hold undertones of a less than satisfactory school report. "Could do better" or "Moments of greatness but tends to get by with the minimum of effort". I was inspired. I was intrigued. I was ready for some research of my own.

The man in my life thought all his Christmases had come at once (whilst I was busy trying to come twice). Out went the oversized T-shirt; on went the stockings, suspenders, and the French maid's outfit. Oui monsieur, non monsieur, three bags full, monsieur. I dusted off the porn, blew cobwebs off the neglected vibrator and went shopping for some fresh surprises. I bent over backwards (literally) in the name of research. If it said do it on a train, we did it on a train. Planes, trains, in the rain, cars, bars, on the stairs, with teddy bears, out loud, extremely proud – Dr Seuss would be happy to declare, we did it almost everywhere.

I began to bore my friends. Sex was all I could talk about and I questioned everyone I met. Then I would race home to test out their theories. In short, it was a sexually-thrilling refresher course. I had become lazy and forgotten what a fun, free, fab way it was to spend time. The more you get, the more you want and I could barely wait to get my kit off. Thankfully, I recovered sufficiently from exhaustion to compile everything in this book.

So whether your sex life is non-existent, fairly flat or downright fabulous there will be something in this book for everyone. Real life stories, how-to's and how-not-to's, hard facts, fun bits and a whole lot more.

So don't just lie there and think of England. Get out there and make sex thrilling and fulfilling. Your partner will be more than willing to join in if you guide them to the bits in the book that will drive you wild (and help you get to the finishing line first). And if you don't have a partner, then flip to the section on doing it for yourself. Because being home alone doesn't mean going without. Been there, done that, got the smile to prove it.

I urge you to embrace this book and all that lies between its covers. You'll be under yours in no time!!

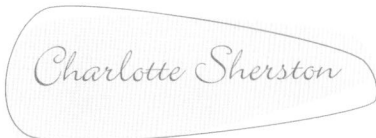

Charlotte Sherston

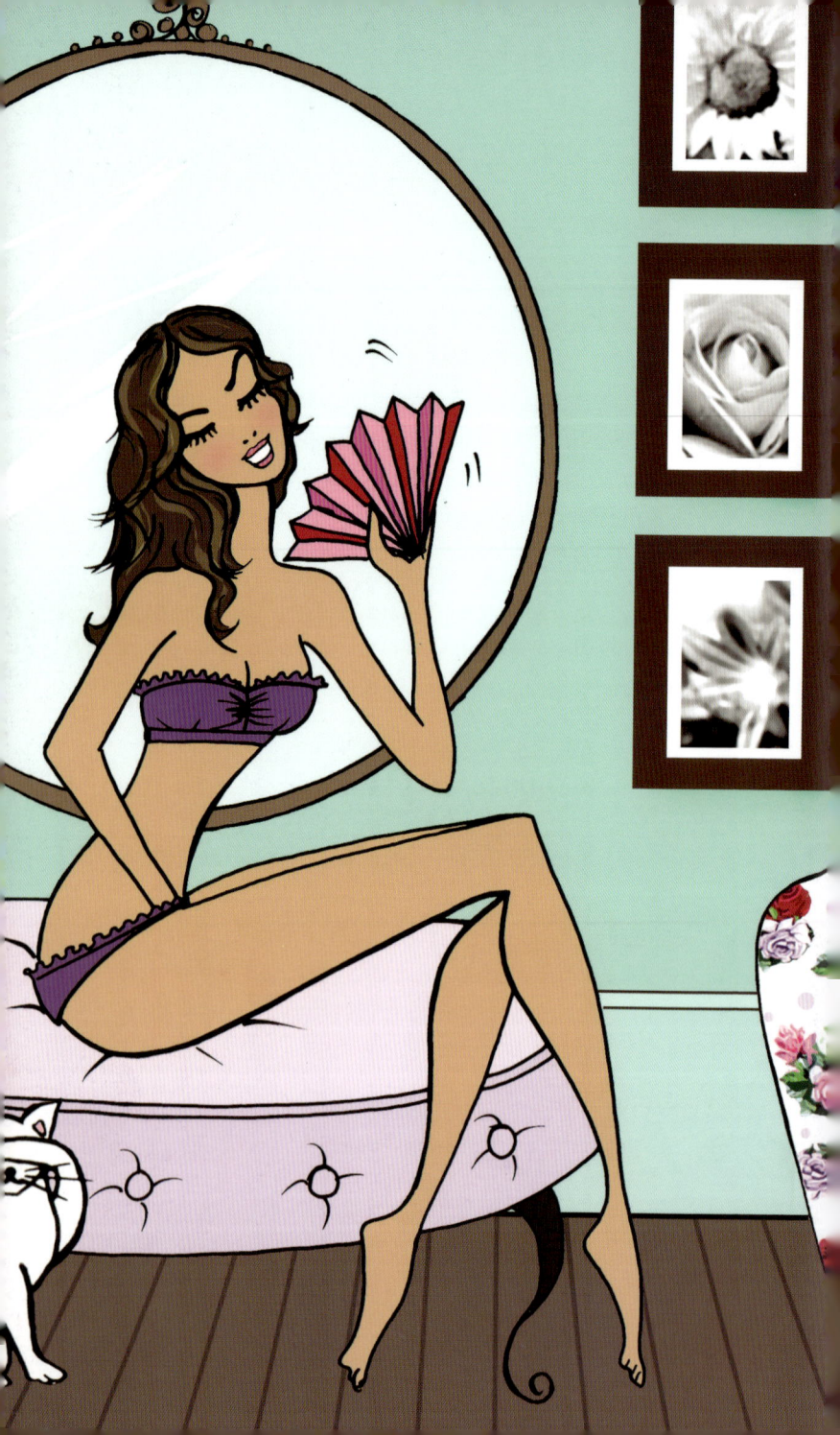

CHAPTER ONE

'The Sound of One Hand...'

THE DIY GUIDE TO MASTURBATION

CHAPTER ONE

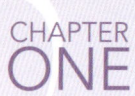

THIS WAS THE ONE THING I DIDN'T TALK ABOUT FOR A LONG TIME. EVEN RECENTLY, IT WAS ONLY IN HUSHED TONES TO CLOSE FRIENDS. WELL OKAY, ONE FRIEND - AND ONLY BECAUSE SHE ASKED. I ALWAYS THOUGHT IT WAS FOR PEOPLE SO DESPERATE THEY HAD TO DO IT THEMSELVES, WHO COULDN'T GET LUCKY SO CONSOLED THEMSELVES WITH A QUICK FUMBLE IN THE PRIVACY OF THEIR OWN HOME.

And then I tried it for myself and ... WHOA! This gave a whole knew meaning to being home alone and having an early night. Early night? I barely left the house. How could it have taken me so long to discover this secret? Who was doing it? Was He? Was She? And why the hell did no-one tell me? If only I had discovered it earlier I probably wouldn't have wasted my time dating half the duds I did. I'd have just kept myself satisfied and saved myself a lot of heartache (Yes, Martin the Bastard, Nick the Juggler and Greg the Dentist - I mean you!)

Aside from the whole fabulous self-satisfaction thing, it's a great way to find out how your body works. And once you

'THE SOUND OF ONE HAND...'

know what rings your bell you can guide any visitor in the right direction. Ding-Dong! Even if you don't have a partner, help is at hand. Yours. Masturbation is a fun, free way to get yourself off without worrying what to wear.

So here's your self-service guide to making yourself one very satisfied customer. Let your fingers do the walking...

WHO IS DOING IT?

Well, obviously, I am. And maybe you are too. If you are, you're in good company: one third of the Australian women surveyed for the book Doing It Down Under have masturbated in the past year, while 20 per cent have indulged in self-pleasuring in the past four weeks, say the book's authors Juliet Richards and Chris Rissel.

If anything masturbation is on the increase and it's certainly not falling out of fashion. It was once believed that self-pleasure was a sure route to insanity ... and now it just seems we're mad for it. So what's changed? Well, one factor is feminism: in addition to pushing for equality in the home, in the classroom and in the workplace, it has advocated for changes in the bedroom. More than any other movement, it's stressed the importance of female pleasure and has brought to attention aspects of sex - such as the G-spot, orgasms and foreplay - that we now take for granted. It gave us permission to explore our own bodies and, by doing so, brought us to the somewhat startling realisation that we could try before we buy. Which comes in very handy!

CHAPTER ONE

WHY DO WE DO IT?

Well, obviously, it feels good ... really, really good. Masturbation is sex. If you believe you're only being sexual when you're with a partner, you're missing out on an entirely satisfying, fulfilling aspect of your sexual self.

Apart from the obvious, masturbation has many other added benefits. It relieves stress, alleviates period pains and helps you get a good night's sleep. Much like yoga but it's more exciting and you don't have to wear scary exercise clothes in front of a full-length mirror. It's healthy, natural and gives your self-confidence and self esteem a boost. And it gets the serotonin pumping, tones up those pelvic floor muscles and instantly puts you in a good mood. Been there, done that ... got the smile to prove it.

By allowing yourself to explore your sexual responses in depth and detail you learn more about your body and what turns you on. Sex therapists and many other health professionals often prescribe masturbation to women who find it hard to orgasm or are experiencing sexual dysfunction. So don't feel guilty ... you're only following doctor's orders.

So, whether you're alone or in a relationship, or somewhere in between, a bit of personal petting is a wonderful, safe way to eliminate sexual tension. Thus avoiding any need to go home with the first guy you meet just because you're horny as hell. Definitely not recommended.

'THE SOUND OF ONE HAND...'.

HOW DO WE DO IT?

Firstly, I think it's important to look at what we're working with (biologically speaking).

Our "pink bits" can be a bit daunting to the uninitiated so it's worth knowing where everything is and how it all works.

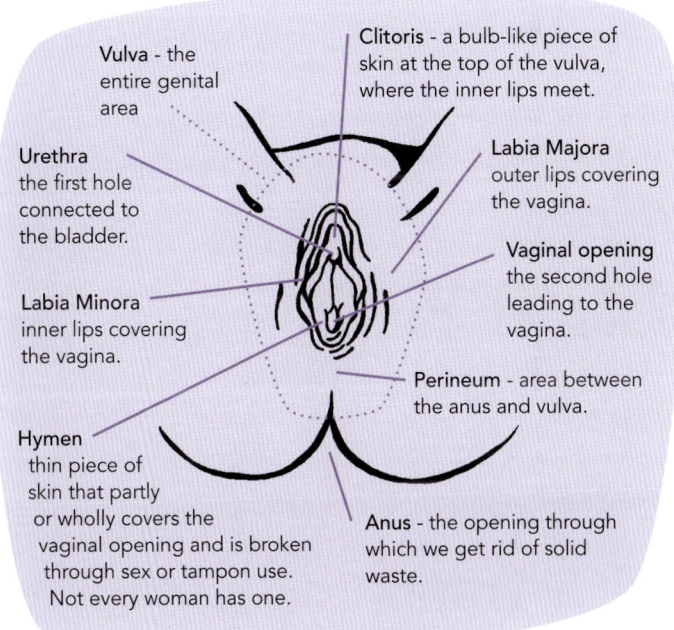

Secondly, the way I do it may be nothing like they way you do (or might do when you give it a shot). When sex researcher Alfred Kinsey surveyed masturbation techniques as part of his landmark work in the '50s, he found the most commonly used techniques by women were:

CHAPTER ONE

- Stimulating the clitoris and inner labia with one or two fingers (the hot favourite).
- Rubbing the outer labia and whole genital area, using the fingers or hand.
- Rhythmically contracting the muscles inside the vagina to simulate intercourse.
- Stimulating the nipples by squeezing them or brushing them lightly with the palms of the hands.
- Vaginal penetration with fingers or objects.

Shere Hite, in later studies of sexual behaviour, found a sixth common masturbation technique: focusing a jet of warm water onto the genital area (for all you fans of the jacuzzi).

GETTING STARTED

Start with whatever you feel comfortable doing; it may be lying on your back, legs wide open, your bottom propped up on a couple of cushions; or lying face down, with a pillow between your legs; or relaxing in your favourite chair watching an erotic video. You might want to stroke yourself lightly through silky underwear; use your fingertips, the pads of your fingers, or your palm (firmly or use a feather light touch). You may prefer indirect clitoral stimulation (the thrill of anticipation can never be underestimated). You might find it arousing to penetrate your vagina/anus with your finger, a dildo or a suitably shaped vegetable (my favourite being the wholesomely thick cucumber). Many women like trickling water on to their vulva or clitoris. Others want to get up on all

'THE SOUND OF ONE HAND…'.

fours and reach a hand or vibrator between their legs while gazing back into a rear positioned mirror. (This is not one for those with "bum look big in this?" issues.)

Take things slowly and don't just go for the obvious erogenous zones first; experiment with pressure and speed and don't forget the largest sexual organ is the brain. Exploring your fantasies is another bonus to personal pleasuring. It's fun to think of something and seeing if it turns you on. Even if it seems weird, warped or banal, go with it and see where it leads. The mental side of masturbation can be as mild or wild, as you want. Even if your thoughts are bizarre, there's no need for alarm, they're only fantasies. Anything goes when it's a walk on the wild side of your imagination.

And the great thing is you don't have to lie there thinking, "Is this right? Is this wrong? Am I about to come? What if I don't? Why didn't I shave my legs this morning?'

You can just relax and enjoy. Half the fun is finding out exactly what turns YOU on most. And what comes a very close second, third and fourth …

HOW DOES SHE DO IT?

Let's be honest, even though it's a very personal thing, we still have an urge to know what other women do. I love a few details, if only for the spark of recognition that often comes with peeping into the private life of others. So in the interest of research we got some busy women to 'fess up to what they do in the comfort of their boudoirs.

CHAPTER ONE

"I slowly massage the lips of my vagina and then, when I feel really excited, I put two of my fingers on either side of my clitoris and squeeze, then move them up and down so the clitoris slides in its hood."

Jacki, 27

"My favourite method is either a hand or a vibrator on my clitoris. I also like to masturbate in a spa with the water jet hitting my vagina."

Monique, 30

"I strip naked, lie on the bed, then warm myself up by playing with my nipples, rubbing my thighs and fingering myself until I am wet. Then I use a dildo to fill up my vagina and at the same time use a vibrator to play with my clitoris."

Anne Marie, 25

(quite the multi-tasker!)

"I use the detachable shower head to directly stimulate my clitoris. I vary the water pressure to change the sensation."

Monique, 21

"Lying on my back with my legs as tight as possible, I gently tickle my clitoris with one bent finger."

Simone, 26

Repeat after me: there is no "right way". Only the right way for you. An undervalued, oft forgotten, mainly hidden way to put a smile on your dial.

'THE SOUND OF ONE HAND...'.

HOW DOES HE DO IT?

In a chapter wholly dedicated to the art of masturbation we can't leave out the boys. If you looked into how many slang words there are for wanking (over 560 at last count) you'd think it was a totally male dominated sport. So whether they are knuckle shuffling, spanking the monkey or choking the chicken, one thing for sure is they are doing it. A lot.

How to masturbate him

Although he's happy to do the job himself he'd be delighted for you to do the honours.

One way to masturbate a man is to try to recreate the feeling of intercourse. The basic idea is to use your hand to simulate the tightness and warmth of the vagina and pump up and down-the strength of your grip depends on his personal preference.

Using a bit of lubricant or saliva, place one or both hands around the erect penis and stroke up and down along the shaft. Some men enjoy the feeling of having the head of their penis encircled with each stroke. As he approaches orgasm, your movements should become more rapid but as he ejaculates, slow down or even stop the pumping action (the head of the penis becomes very sensitive at this stage).

CHAPTER ONE

It is generally proclaimed that men think about sex every seven minutes, so you can hardly blame the poor lads for having their hands in their pants at every opportunity.

Unlike us they usually feel less guilt and tend to be far more open about it with their mates. Like us, they occasionally use props; creams, oils, gels, fruit, pies, gloves or simply swap hands for a bit of variety. A visual aid is a popular choice too: music videos, girls' mags (such as CLEO), porn mags, porn films ... porn of any kind really.

Fantasies range from the usual suspects - Britney/Christina/Kylie - to their ex, the hot girl at the office, their flatmate's sister, the girl next door ... they could be thinking about anyone really. Except you. Current girlfriends, lovers or wives seldom appeared on the Top Ten.

DICK*tionary*

Hand shandy *n. A frothy one, pulled off the wrist*
Vinegar strokes *n. The final, climatic stages of male masturbation. As in, "Would you believe it? The phone rang just as I was getting onto the vinegar strokes." From the similar facial expressions achieved when sipping vinegar.*
Wanking spanners *n. hands*

'THE SOUND OF ONE HAND…'.

Props

Sex toys of all shapes and sizes can be used for further enjoyment or additional help reaching orgasm. See Chapter 7 for a fabulously detailed look at all the options. But remember that household objects can give varied erotic sensations too. Just use your imagination. Try these for starters:

- Feathers, feather boas
- Strings of pearls/beads/fine chains (watch the clasps)
- Silk or chiffon scarves
- Velvet
- Scented oils
- Candles/candle wax
- Zucchinis, cucumbers, carrots, grapes or strawberries
- Electric toothbrushes
- Ice cubes
- Whipped cream

Some women find it hard to understand why he still feels the need to wank when he is getting regular sex. In the eloquent words of Oliver, 30,

"Convenience. I don't have to wait for my hand to be 'in the mood'. I don't have to take it out for dinner and pay it compliments. I don't worry that my hand will become jealous and tell me to 'stop looking at that other hand'. If I want some action, it's right there without any hassles."

Dave, 22, goes a small way toward redeeming his race by adding, "It's definitely a case of only doing it when the girlfriend isn't there. The feeling isn't comparable to having sex with her-no way! I'd take the girl over my hand any day." (Well, good for you Dave ... I hope you're girlfriend would do the same for you.)

So what are you waiting for? Go home and explore! And next time you're wondering if your prince will come, you'll know you can get there before he does.

A WORD ABOUT GUILT AND SHAME.

Isn't it ironic that we're all quite happy to talk endlessly and graphically, about shape, size, fit, taste and technique but will rarely mention a solo session in all-girl company?

"It's embarrassing," says Lisa, a 26-year-old graphic designer. "Sure, I own a vibrator and when my boyfriend's out I'll use it on myself but I keep it well hidden from him and he has absolutely no idea of what I get up to when he's not here - I'm pretty sure he'd be shocked. But it's not like I've told my girlfriends either. It's still such a taboo area as far as women are concerned."

Even in these sexually sophisticated times, we're not always as cool and liberated as we'd like to be. Some of us were brought up in times or in cultures where masturbation, if not considered downright sinful, was certainly a subject not fit for public consideration and discussion - it was something to be kept secret. And a number of us were "caught in the act" as children and punished, teased or humiliated as a

'THE SOUND OF ONE HAND…'.

consequence. Such conditioning can be difficult to shake but thousands manage it and you can too. I have to restrain myself when my own daughter (five and quite fascinated by the human body) insists on flashing her knickers and having a fiddle in front of company. God forbid I give her a lifetime complex!

Please remember you aren't doing anything wrong - you are having safe, adult sex in total privacy (I hope anyway … privacy is best for all concerned; I did explain that to my daughter). If you find it difficult, despite your efforts, to relax and enjoy masturbation think about getting a professional to help. Sex therapists have many effective techniques at their disposal for helping people come to terms with their sexuality and success is usually speedy and lasting.

For information on sex therapy and counselling contact ASSERT (Australian Society of Sex Educators, Researchers and Therapists) on (02) 9280 0151; or the Australian Psychological Society on 1800 333 497.

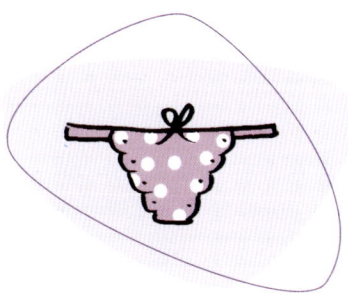

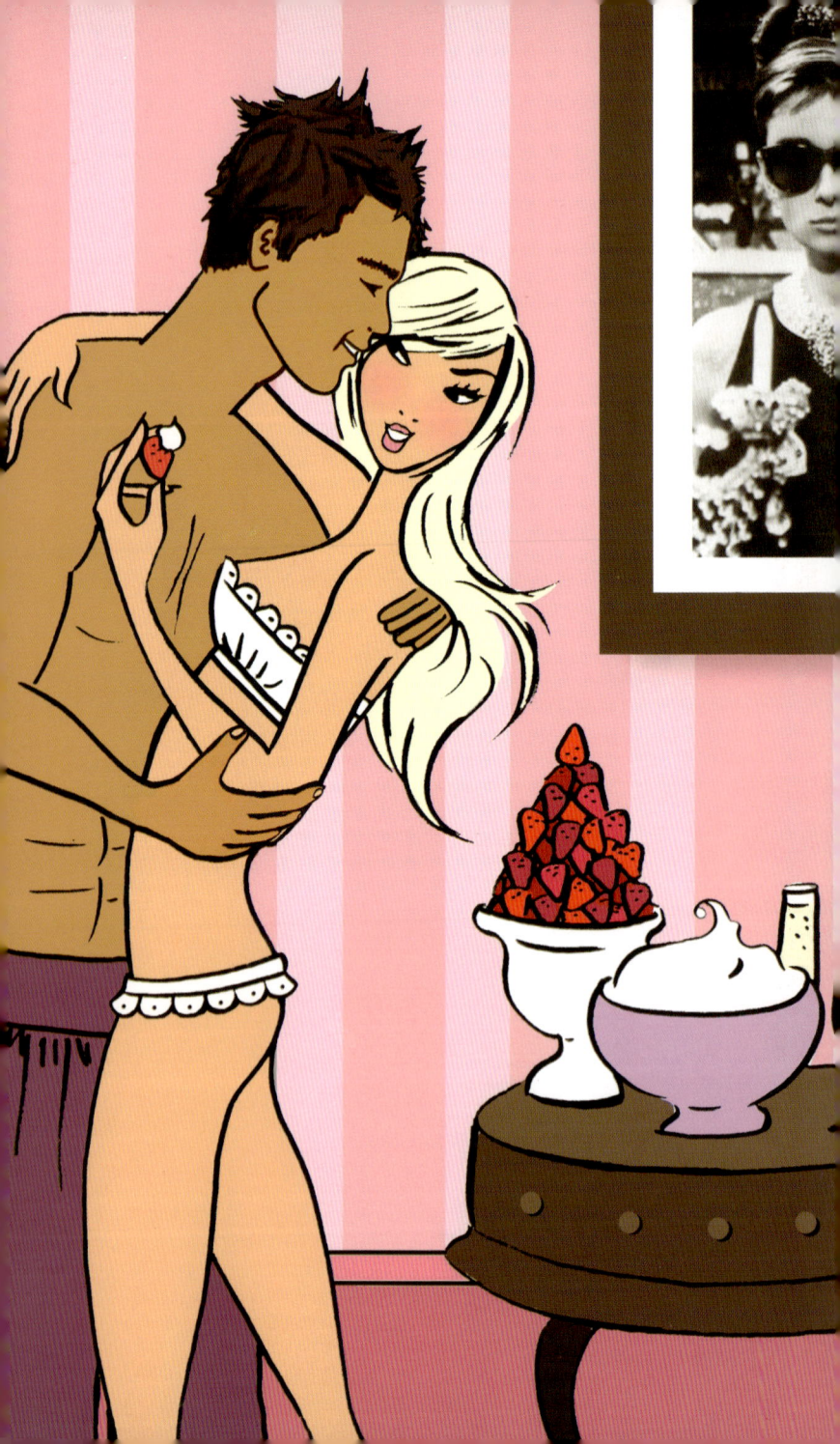

CHAPTER TWO

How to Get Your Engine Started

FOREPLAY

CHAPTER TWO

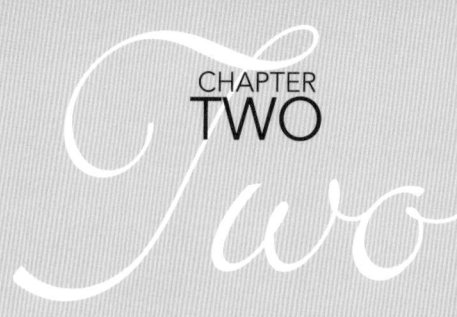

LACK OF FOREPLAY IS RARELY A MALE COMPLAINT. IN FACT YOU GET THE FEELING THAT MOST OF THEM WOULD HAPPILY SIDE STEP THE WARM UP COMPLETELY AND JUST GO STRAIGHT TO THE MAIN EVENT. WE GIRLS TAKE A BIT MORE TIME TO GET OUR ENGINE STARTED. SOMETIMES IT WOULD TAKE A TEAM OF MECHANICS TO GET MINE HUMMING ALONG (NOTE TO SELF: ADD TEAM OF MECHANICS TO FANTASY HOT LIST).

This disparity is a great shame. Because foreplay is half the fun: the build up, the add-ons, the sheer anticipation is part of what makes sex so fabulous. And if you are still a virgin or in a new relationship foreplay is the action. There are plenty of things you can do without getting your knickers off that would put a smile on both your faces. You can still have great sex without intercourse. And as only 33 per cent of women orgasm through penetration alone, that leaves 67 per cent of you absolutely panting for some more first course.

The aim of this chapter is to remind you to slow down and have a little patience. Let us show you how you can make a whole night of it and play games where everyone's a winner. Learn new twists on old faves. And hopefully introduce him

HOW TO GET YOUR ENGINE STARTED

to the merits of delayed gratification. A little less wham-bam will do you the world of good and get your engine purring nicely.

FOREPLAY - WHAT IS IT?

Also known as "outercourse", "almost sex" or "everything but", it can encompass kissing, cuddling, genital stimulation and frottage (rubbing against each other with your clothes on). Basically anything that gets you turned on except intercourse. So, it covers a whole lot of good stuff that is sadly overlooked a lot of the time. Highly recommended for everyone and a prerequisite for most.

SEX WITH YOUR CLOTHES ON (well, almost....)

There's something oh-so delicious about anticipation. So instead of stampeding in for the grand finale, check out our guide to erotic foreplay. Tease your man right and you'll have him begging for more.

MOVE #1
Dirty Dialling
Great sex engages all the senses but few people give credit to its verbal component. With a single call you can send your man into a frenzy of excitement and leave him sitting at his desk with a hard on and a head full of wicked thoughts. And this way, he'll be thinking about you and not the cute girl at reception!

Dr Gabrielle Morrissey, head of the Sexology Program at Curtin University in Perth, suggests that "before you call, pick your tone: flirty, seductive, romantic, vampy, dominatrix."

CHAPTER TWO

When he answers, stay silent for a few seconds. Then in your sexiest voice, describe how you'd like him to kiss you, touch you and undress you. Then take him through the finer details of how you are going to give him the most amazing oral sex ever. "Non-verbal communication is a good element too," adds Dr Morrissey. "You can groan and moan, but you can also breathe, stay silent and then tell him what you just did to yourself." This may be just pouring a cup of tea or checking your emails but he doesn't need to know that.

A word of warning too, from someone who tends to trip up at any given opportunity. Phone sex is best when he isn't about to rush off to a class or a meeting. He'll be distracted for all the wrong reasons. And listen closely for the subtle clues that tell you that you're on loudspeaker. In an early attempt at debauched dialling I was stopped mid groan by a stifled chuckle. The man in question didn't tell me he was with six mates. Hot and bothered? You betcha.

MOVE #2
Mouth to Mouth

Remember when you were still a teenager and you kissed until you got stubble rash? Don't underestimate the power of the pash now you're all grown up. Get cosy on the couch without it leading to anything else (and, yes, that means no hand up your top.) "Try kissing around the edges of the lips, then run the tip of your tongue over the gums," says Nitya Lacroix, author of The Complete Guide To Sexual Fulfilment. "The longer you can delay before inserting your tongue, the more sensual it will be. Lift his face and teasingly kiss him around the chin and jaw, moving down to the sensitive areas of the neck and throat."

HOW TO GET YOUR ENGINE STARTED

If you really can't resist taking your tongues further afield, extend your pash to a 'tongue bath' (which feels much nicer than it sounds!), where you cover every inch of your lover's body with kisses. Blindfold him if it takes your fancy, then make him lie still while you go to work caressing and nibbling.

MOVE # 3
Have a clothes encounter

Another nostalgic trip back to teenage times when you rubbed up against each other so hard you could have started a campfire. Nowadays, when nakedness seems to be the norm, doing it clothed can deliver a certain illicit thrill. The "dry hump" (why do all these tantalising activities sound so awful?) re-creates that feeling when you thought you'd go crazy if he didn't get it inside you right now. The advantage is that, this time, your dad is unlikely to walk in on you.

MOVE # 4
Feeding frenzy

Bearing in mind that men find women with healthy appetites sexy as hell, what more deliciously appropriate place to unleash your inner seductress than at a restaurant? While you're reading the menu, play footsies with him under the table. Lick your lips, suck the strawberry in your champers and take his hand in yours, stroking his fingers up and down, simulating what you would like to do with his penis. Seriously, it sounds unsubtle and it is. But men are simple creatures at heart - have you watched any porn? Nothing subtle about it at all.

CHAPTER TWO

MOVE #5
Get your kit off

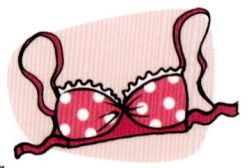

All right, for this one, you do get to take your clothes off. The crucial maxim when stripping for someone is to forget about being self-conscious. Trust us, he isn't going to think you're an idiot when he's getting his own private striptease - especially when he's got a front row seat and he anticipates he'll be gettin' some afterwards. Remember you're the prize, so peel off each layer sensually and s-l-o-w-l-y. Set the scene by playing some sexy music and tease away. Swivel your hips in a figure eight motion and walk with one foot directly in front of the other. Take a feather boa or scarf and run it across your shoulders, arching your back (that's right, stick your chest out!). With your back to him, shrug the jacket off your shoulders and then remove one sleeve at a time but don't let it go! Turn to face him, and then remove one hand at a time, allowing it to drop. Next, unzip your skirt, let it fall and leave it on the floor. Now kick off your shoes. Undo your bra clasp, pull it out from under your

> *"We don't want sex to be routine. My boyfriend and I waited until we couldn't take it any longer before we finally had sex. Now we'll sometimes go without intercourse for a week. I'm a romantic. I don't want it to be ordinary."*
>
> *Diane, 26*

HOW TO GET YOUR ENGINE STARTED

arms, and then slide it away, stroking your nipples. Place your palms inside the sides of your knickers and lift them away from your body. Step out delicately, one foot at a time. It's showtime!

Top tip: A glass of vino and a trial run are recommended for those not naturally swan-like.

MOVE #6
Make a clean shave of it

There's nothing like getting dirty while staying clean. Invite him to join you in a great big bubble bath. Work up a soapy lather on his back, write secret messages on his skin and ask him to guess what they are. Shampoo his hair and massage his feet. Begin to shave your legs, then pass him the razor (not one for those of you with trust issues) and get him to shave even more. By the time he's done, your bath won't be the only thing frothing over.

MOVE #7
Slow hand

Trusty tome *The Joy Of Sex* sings the praises of a technique called "spider's legs", which involves massage aiming to stimulate not so much the skin as the almost invisible skin hairs. "The essence is in the extreme lightness of touch - more electric that tickling," according to the sex manual by Alex Comfort. "Use both hands, keep a steady progression of movements going with one and make surprise attacks with the other." Don't lunge for the genitals (take note three-quarters of the male species!), instead focus on the most sensitive areas - neck, chest, nipples, belly, arms, thighs, back, palms, scrotum and perineum.

CHAPTER TWO

MOVE #8
Lap it up.....
All the thrills of his own lap-dancer without any need to whip his wallet out. When I tried this one at home I felt it only fair that I did get a few dollars for my trouble, but you may be a better woman than I. Slick on a little baby oil to give your body a sexy sheen and take him to the edge by letting him get as close as he dares without touching. Get him to sit down, while you wiggle your crotch just a tongue's length away. Maintain eye contact while you touch yourself. And if he does try to touch you? Slap away the naughty boy's hand.

MOVE #9
Give great hand.
Our bodies have thousands of nerve endings, so hands can create hours of non-stop sexual stimulation.

We asked sexpert Lou Paget, author of *365 Days Of Sensational Sex*, for these must-know moves.

Before you begin make sure you:
- Lubricate or, at the very least, moisten the area with saliva before you start.
- Practice on a dildo, a cucumber or a willing partner (who unlike a vegetable can give you feedback!)
- Ask him to masturbate in front of you if you're not sure what he likes.

HOW TO GET YOUR ENGINE STARTED

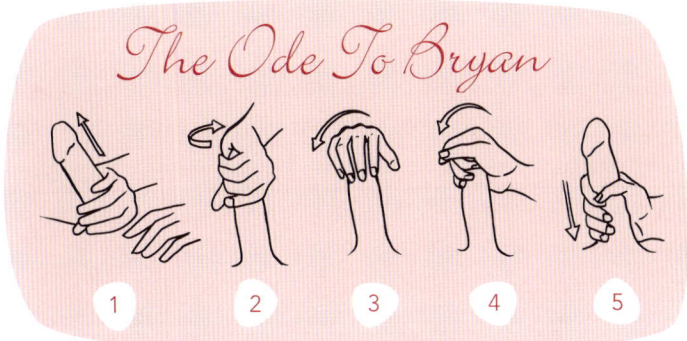

The Ode To Bryan

1. Facing your partner, start with your hands in front of you, thumbs down. You should be looking at the back of your hand and four fingers. His view would be of your thumb nestled in his pubic hair. Position your other hand so it's ready to take over from the first when you've completed one cycle. Stroke up the penis in a single and continuos motion.
2. When you've reached the head, twist your hand slightly, as if you were carefully opening a jar.
3. Maintain as much contact as possible; rotate your hand over the top of the penis.
4. Your thumb will now be facing you and the back of your hand will be facing him. Move firmly over the top of the penis.
5. Move down the shaft to the base. Immediately shift your second hand in to position on top of your first hand. There should be a continuos flow of sensations; when one hand stops the other hand takes over. You'll get the flow of motion very quickly. Alternate hands repeatedly. Eventually just focus on the movements at the head of the penis.

CHAPTER TWO

MOVE #10
Special request

Tell your lover that for one night only, you're going to be his sex slave. Present him with some blank cards on which he writes down the things he'd like you to do to him - anything goes, except the act. He shuffles them; you pick one and perform the request written on it. However, it's crucial you're comfortable with his request too. Good foreplay is all about getting turned on in the build up to orgasmic sex, so don't do anything you don't want to. And remember, even though you might feel a bit silly dressed up in the bunny girl outfit, smile, because it's his turn next.

BLOW HIM AWAY

This deserved a section all its own.

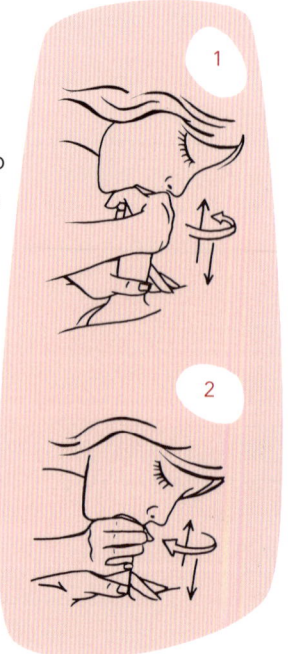

I was hard pressed to find a man who didn't rate oral sex as his favourite forerunner. Most were stunned that a woman was even suggesting ways to be better at it - they were just happy to get it at all and thought that a bad blow job seemed a contradiction in terms. One did sheepishly admit that he always told girls that he didn't like blow jobs. As a result they were down on their knees in no time trying to change his mind (who said women

HOW TO GET YOUR ENGINE STARTED

had the monopoly on manipulation!). However, if you get this bit right, you will rise to the rank of ultimate sex goddess. But don't forget you get plenty of brownie points just for trying.

Blow-by-Blow account.
"Give him front row action by tying your hair back," says Tracey Cox in *Supersex*. "And lick your way downwards until his penis is straining for attention. Then bypass it by licking down the outside of his inner thigh to his testicles. Stop there and drive him nuts using tongue movements to swirl round each one." The secret to a mind numbing blow job is variety. Use a range of elements and vary the speed and intensity of your movements. It doesn't need to be complicated - just do what feels good to your mouth.

It's all in the technique
Up and down: With your hand "sealed" to your mouth, move up and down the length of the shaft, varying the length and speed of the stroke. Adjust the amount of pressure by opening your mouth wider.

Twist: Rotate the sealed hand back and forth.

Tongue magic: Keen for something new? Put two fingers together inside your mouth and move your tongue all around them, keeping it moving as you slide your fingers in and out. The same effect works just as well on his testicles.

Teabagging: Drive him wild by dipping his balls in to your mouth. If you're feeling brave, try both at once.

CHAPTER TWO

DO:
- Stroke the perineum (skin between his testicles and anus)
- Keep your tongue in motion constantly
- Look at him-most men are 'suckers' for this.

DON'T
- Leave your teeth exposed. This can be very painful for him.
- Try to deep throat before you are ready.
- Suck hard just after he's come. The head of the penis is at its most sensitive straight after ejaculation.

With the average penis larger than the average mouth, it doesn't take a rocket scientist to work out some of the shaft's going to be left out in the cold. The answer? Hands-on action. Make a ring around the base of the penis with your fingers while sucking on the end. "If you are going to gag (never a good look), change position," says Cox. "Get him to stand while you sit on the bed facing him. Use one hand to control his penis and now you are in the perfect position to control how deeply you take him in.

HARD ACT TO SWALLOW

Fellatio is one thing, but it's what comes after that has us much divided. Assuming you know it's not high in kilojoules (it's protein, not fat), and assuming you've discovered there's only one innocuous tablespoonful (which still represents enough sperm to populate the whole of China) what's a gulp between friends? Apparently a lot. Oral sex is a normal activity for 88 per cent of men and 87 per cent of women, according to a recent report, but that's where agreement ends. What's physiologically a dribble is psychologically a

HOW TO GET YOUR ENGINE STARTED

torrent to many women. Here's what they had to say on the subject (I can still see the grimaces now).

"Whoever said it tasted like a combination of buttermilk and bleach was on target."

Rachel, 29

"Swallowing makes me feel violated. It's as if he's putting something over me, like, 'Ha! You swallowed."

Lisa, 26

"I always swallow. It's a turn on to see how much pleasure he gets from it."

Lisa, 33

"A great big yuck is all I have to say on the subject."

Anita, 28

And the boys….

"What's the point if you're not going to swallow? To me, it's like going down on a girl and only going halfway. I think you should give it 100% whether you are a guy or girl"

Mark, 30

"If guys could do it themselves-and most have tried unsuccessfully-they would swallow for one reason alone: not having to clean it up."

Liam, 25

"Spitting is not good. If chicks really object to the taste, then take him out before he climaxes and let him come on your body."

James, 27

CHAPTER TWO

"I think it's the biggest turn on ever if a girl swallows. Plain and simple. Maybe it's animal instinct."
Graham, 28

"I don't care - I should be thanking her for letting me near her mouth. What's the policy there anyhow? Do you tell her you are just about to blow or just do it and hope for the best? There should be some sort of etiquette!"
Greg, 29

" A satisfied swallow is a fitting conclusion to a very giving act, while spitting simply represents rejection."
Fraser, 30

To swallow or not to swallow? YOU DECIDE

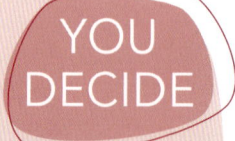

- What's in a gulp? In a single ejaculation, semen usually consists of 200,000 - 300,000 sperm and contains citric acid, sodium, zinc, potassium and enzymes. It can also contain fat and protein.
- Full of flavour? If the taste of your partner's semen is your main gripe when it comes to swallowing, there's a way to change it. Sweeten the taste of his ejaculate by getting him to drink pineapple juice.
- Is it fattening? The average ejaculate contains 151 kilojoules - that's equal to eating 10 pistachio nuts.
- How long does it take? About 83 per cent of me climax in less than five minutes.
- Endless supply? The average man ejaculates 18 litres of semen during his lifetime.

HOW TO GET YOUR ENGINE STARTED

Are you sensing a theme here? Most men love it and most women are less than keen. Alarmingly, no-one mentioned the issue that should be uppermost in everybody's mind. Inger, an AIDS educator agrees, "The question isn't should you swallow, but why do you have a penis in your mouth that doesn't have a condom on it?" Although few cases of AIDS have been linked to fellatio, an HIV-infected man does carry the virus in his semen and its transmission is possible through genital-oral contact if sores or cuts are present in the mouth. So if you don't know his HIV status - use a condom.

For those of us in monogamous relationships with HIV-negative partners the swallow debate rages on. Everyone agreed that a gentleman should give a lady fair warning when he's coming so she has a choice. As for men who want their women to swallow, one suggestion: consider your diet. Different men taste differently, so if you're doing lots of smoking, drinking and drugs, your partner is literally going to taste your lifestyle, and that taste may not be pleasant. The key issue seems to be the male ego (bless them), with many men regarding your choice as a reflection of your feelings for him. So if you are not keen to ingest his offering, try to avoid: 1) Running straight to the sink. 2) Gagging in dramatic fashion. 3) Muttering something like "Have you eaten anchovies lately?"

Imagine how you would feel if he behaved similarly after pleasuring you downstairs. Best bet is to hold it in your mouth (he'll think you swallowed and that you are amazing), then subtly spit it into your hand and dispose of it in sink/on towel/etc. Trust us, he'll never forget you.

CHAPTER TWO

GAMES –GET SET TO GET OFF.

I am a huge fan of games, despite being an uncharitable loser. The good thing about these bedroom games is their win-win element. Not recommended for an afternoon with the relatives around ... these are strictly for behind closed doors.

The Fitness Assessment You need: Rope, an egg timer, pens and paper. How to play: both write lists of different body parts on separate pieces of paper, fold them up and scatter them over the bed. One of you gets tied up, the other picks a folded up note. Focus all your energy on the body part written down until the timer runs out. Take turns.

Spin the bottle You need: A bottle and a flat surface to spin it on. How to play: This game is all about getting in the mood. Sit opposite each other on the floor or at a table. Place the bottle in the centre and spin it to decide who goes first. Whoever the top of the bottle points to should start by making up the first sentence of an erotic story. Check out www.cleansheets.com for inspiration. Then take turns to spin the bottle and add a sentence to build up your sexy tale.

Slippery Dip You need: Slippery Sex Sheets with Neon Body Paints ($35.95 available through www.adultshop.com.au) Includes a protective mat and scented, squirtable body paint. How to play: To loosen up your muscles, get into some messy foreplay. Then, spread the protective sheet on the bed and choose your preferred colour paint. Then take it in turns to mould each other into position and use your

HOW TO GET YOUR ENGINE STARTED

partner's body as a canvas. The best part? Messing up your masterpiece. When the paint runs out, honey or chocolate sauce make a yummy substitute.

The Cool Factor You need: ice, towels, champagne and a hot bath. How to play: Run a hot bath, place folded tea towels at either end and pour two glasses of bubbly. Both climb in the tub and face each other, resting your heads on the towels. Take turns rubbing ice cubes over your partner's body with your fingers or toes. The challenge? To bring the other person to orgasm by turning them on with the ice.

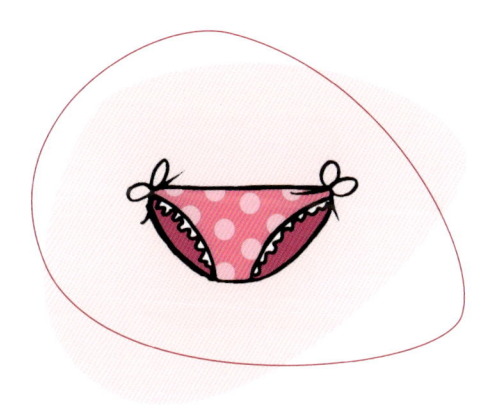

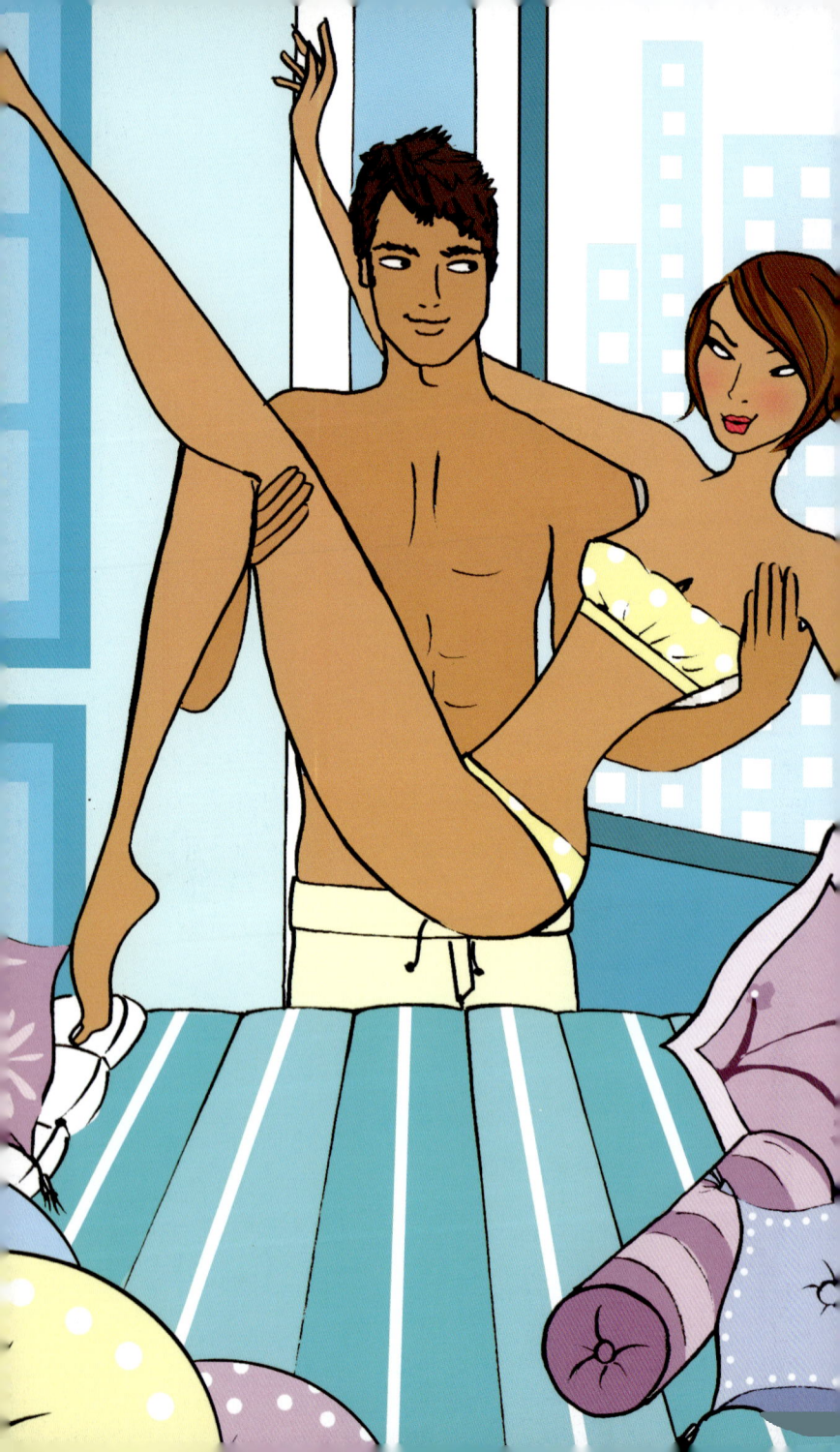

CHAPTER THREE

The Main Event

SEX - A BEGINNER'S GUIDE

CHAPTER THREE

IF YOU HAVE DILIGENTLY READ THE CHAPTERS PRECEDING THIS ONE I MUST CONGRATULATE YOU ON YOUR PATIENCE. OF COURSE YOU WILL HAVE LEARNT BY NOW THAT THE ACT OF INTERCOURSE IS BY NO MEANS THE BE ALL AND END ALL. HOWEVER, ALTHOUGH YOU MAY MAKE A FEW DETOURS ALONG THE WAY, YOU EVENTUALLY WILL GET TO YOUR FINAL DESTINATION. "TICKETS PLEASE, LADIES AND GENTLEMEN. NEXT STOP, SEXUAL INTERCOURSE. PLEASE BE SURE TO TAKE ALL YOUR BELONGINGS WITH YOU AND ENJOY THE REST OF THE RIDE."

SHOULD YOU OR SHOULDN'T YOU?

Let's back up just for a moment - in the hope of avoiding any morning-after regrets. There is nothing worse than that grubby feelng of wishing you hadn't had sex with him. There are a couple of things worth considering before you dive between the sheets.

1. Is he single?
More importantly, is he honest about his status? You can make you own decisions about married men without us, but you have the right to know the whole truth and base your

THE MAIN EVENT

decision on that before you step into the great unknown. This is tough on you because it's usually the most outwardly attractive and charming of men who two-time. Men with something to hide take great care in avoiding the issue. A man like this thinks the fact that he's not actually living with his girlfriend of the past three years gives him carte blanche. A man who's attached will drop hints about having "a few very close female friends", and when you ask about how he spends his time, will have lots of things to do like "training", and "visiting his nanna" (early morning relative visiting is highly suspicious at the best of times). This is all fine if you genuinely just want a one-night stand with this individual and are absolutely convinced you will not be waiting around for him to call you tomorrow. Because he won't call you, he'll be busy with someone else.

2. Can you stand anyone else knowing about it?
Sex is never a secret. Especially sex between two interesting, attractive individuals with careers and social lives. Other people will catch on. Both sets of friends may rib you. This is easy to deal with, just refuse to confirm or deny it and keep the details to yourself. If you can't stand anyone else knowing about it at all costs – for instance if you could lose your job, your home or your health over it, or some other devastating consequence we haven't thought of, then think again.

3. Do you feel comfortable with yourself?
You know, all those little things like, are you wearing the right underwear? Has the rash gone from your last bikini wax? We only ask because discomfort over your appearance or

CHAPTER THREE

body can cause a serious lack of self-confidence that may devastate your performance - and thus kill your sexual relationship before it's even begun. Any man worth his salt won't care whether you've shaved under your arms or not, but if the fact that you haven't is going to inhibit your fun, then give it a miss. No girl ever enjoyed sex after she spent ten minutes pointing out her fat bits (it wasn't those bits he was looking at!).

4. Will anyone be hurt?

Be sensible if he is the boyfriend/husband/partner of a friend or family member, if he's the brother of your broken-hearted old flame, if he's the man who broke your bestie's heart last year – think twice. Is it really worth the scandal and the hurt that will ensue? Do you really want this man to be able to closely compare your friend's sexual techniques with yours? If you really feel that you're falling in love and it's not just sex and you can face the fiasco, then go ahead. Good luck.

5. Will the sex be safe?

Look, you shouldn't even have to ask. Take your own supply of condoms and solve the dilemma.

6. Why him?

Why are you contemplating sex with this man? Is it because you genuinely want to make love with him? Or are you simply lonely? We can be in love with the idea of love, especially when we haven't had any for a while. Don't go home with him just for the company, unless you feel completely happy about saying goodbye in the morning. And never seeing him again. Also beware of the rebound – yours or his. If he's broken-hearted, he is only looking for comfort love. If you think you'd like a relationship with him, tell him to come back

THE MAIN EVENT

in six months. If you're on the rebound and missing your ex, you will miss him much more desperately in a bed with someone else.

7. Is there an escape?
Be sure to have an exit route if you change your mind, which you are completely entitled to at any time. A sudden phantom stomach bug or mention of some menstrual-related incident is usually enough to kill the mood and give you a get out.

8. How will you feel the next day?
Bright, bubbly and brilliant? Or dirty and disappointed? Give it some thought and work out if he's worth it.

ABOUT LAST NIGHT

So you did it. Most of us have experienced the thrills and spills of getting down and dirty on the first date. The next day, some of us can't get the smiles off our faces, while others feel more sorry than sexy. But what we want to know is, what are our male counterparts thinking?

"If girls put out on the first date, it's no different to guys who perhaps want the same thing. So ultimately, I really don't think there's anything morally wrong with it." *Joseph, 29*

"I would wonder if there was any future in our involvement, beyond sex, but I certainly wouldn't think any worse of her." *Brent, 35*

"As with most things, you get what you pay for, and if you didn't pay anything it probably won't be worth much." *Len, 37*

CHAPTER THREE

"What I'm looking for in a partner is not someone who gives it up on the first date, but someone who makes me wait – to test my commitment to the overall relationship, and not just the sex."

Jackson, 28

"Put it this way, a guy will not say no to a bonk. But if a girl wants a boy to come back for more, I'd recommend waiting."

Lachlan, 22

"If I've had a few too many, then I'll kind of be hoping she will put out, but otherwise I'm kind of hoping she won't – because if I really like her, I'll be too nervous to perform."

Lee, 22

"My girlfriend picked me up in a bar, took me home and we shagged all night. We've been together for six years."

Michael, 34

"If we've just met in a club or bar and the sexual chemistry is there and she wants to pursue it in the sack, then I'm all for it. I wouldn't think anything bad about her – but the thing is, I probably wouldn't be thinking much about her at all after that."

Anthony, 27

SEX POSITIONS

I've read those books full of every position possible (and a few that are damn near impossible). They are fine if you happen to be a 16-year-old gymnast, which I sadly am not. So, we decided instead to keep it simple. Something old (the classic moves), something new (you may not have tried),

THE MAIN EVENT

something for him and something for you. All explained and illustrated to ensure you'll keep the neighbours awake and envious.

Missionary magic
This is a sexual staple in most people's repertoire. And for good reason. It is terrific for intimacy and very bonding. For a change, bring your legs into play by resting them on his butt. This in turn elevates your pelvis, allowing his pubic bone to gently rub against your clitoris. If you have the desire and hamstrings to carry this off, lift your legs onto his shoulders for penetration that's deep and meaningful. Just remember to take it slowly.

Cat call
Known as CAT (clitoral alignment technique), you assume the missionary position but instead of your man doing the same, he slides a few centimetres forward from where he usually is. He cups your shoulders so his body falls flat against yours. The base of his penis should naturally rub against your clitoris. With your legs straight out, push your pelvis up a bit; he pushes down to provide counter-resistance. Rock gently up and down, instead of in and out. Worth the effort.

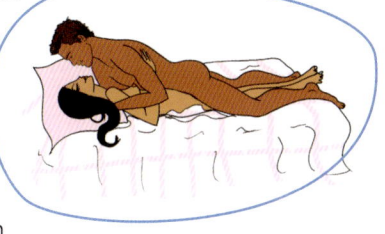

CHAPTER THREE

Ride him, Cowgirl!
Hello G-spot, hello C-spot, hello O hello! For a clitoral orgasm, straddle him, lean your torso forward, arch your back and keep your crotch close to his penis. Now rock. Want a G-gantic climax? Lean back and have him support you with his hands.

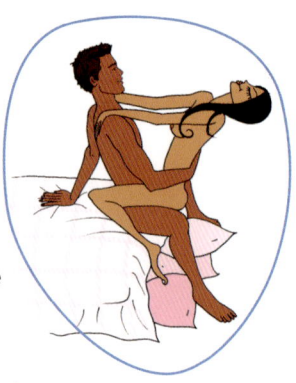

Ruff and Ready
Add a new dimension to doggie style by assuming the standard position but with your knees as close to the edge of the bed as possible, and your hands in front of you. Your man stands behind you, feet on the floor. This results in him having a greater range of movement and he can consequently thrust with more power.

Is this seat taken?
A comfortable way to relax into rear entry sex. Here you control the action while he sits back and relaxes to enjoy the ride. If you want to make it all about him, sit him in a chair and spend a few active moments 'in his lap' then when you are both suitably aroused turn around and gently guide his penis in to your vagina. Sit on him as you would a chair. His hands will be

THE MAIN EVENT

free to rub all over your body or to hold your hips to increase the intensity of penetration. You can then move your hips and have a little wiggle from side to side in rhythm with him or bend forward and leverage support from the floor or his knees if you want a really bouncy ride. Giddy up!

CSI (clit scene investigation)

If you're looking for a penetrative climax (hello, I'll take two) we've found the move. It may sound like an ordinary woman-on-top position, but the slightest modification can make the world of difference. Here your knees become the pivotal point of action. Face and straddle him. Rest your hands on the back of his legs, just above his knees, while he places his hands on your knees and lifts your knees a few centimetres off the bed. With his penis at your vaginal entrance and not very far inside, gently rock back and forth and back and forth and ...The whole point of the exercise? His penis will come out, touching your clitoris as you rock back, and then slide back in as you rock forward.

Sexy snuggle up

The perfect position for lazy lovemaking. Enjoy the intimacy. Lying on your sides facing one another, he enters you with his top leg bent and resting

CHAPTER THREE

between your thighs and his bottom leg straight. Your top leg rests on his side, while your lower leg on the mattress stretches along his. Your pelvis controls the pace; tease him with fast flutters before slowing down to take in the arousal. Side positions are great for women because the way our legs are positioned results in extra stimulation of the labia and thrusts are felt much more deeply.

Dick Racy

This position is win-win; he achieves deep, intense penetration while your clitoris has a little celebration of pleasure too. You lie on your back with your bum at the bed's edge; he enters you from a kneeling position on the floor, gently placing your feet into position - one foot on his chest, the other resting up along his body and over his shoulder. Who said you couldn't have your porn queen moment?

ANAL SEX

I don't know many women who haven't encountered a man trying to slip one in the backdoor like he's simply made a wrong turn. Anal sex used to be taboo but now it's part of the sexual repertoire for many couples. Think you're the only one not doing it?

Nothing divides a room full of women like the subject of anal sex. For some it's the last frontier. For others it's something to try once and then discard. And then there are women who swear by it as one of life's great pleasures.

THE MAIN EVENT

According to The Great CLEO Sex Survey 2003, 47 per cent of you have tried anal sex at least once. However, according to Dr Gabrielle Morrissey, head of Sexology at Perth's Curtin University, "anal eroticism is 'on the menu' more than it ever was. People are definitely more curious about anal sex – even if they're not actively experimenting with it.

What a boy wants
Since anal sex is usually thought to be forbidden, this can be a turn-on for some. "The thrill of breaking a taboo can take us back to when we discovered sex for the first time," says Dr Morrissey.

Men also cite a different physical sensation as one of the reasons they're drawn to it. "The external sphincter is very tight," says Dr Morrissey. "Some men argue that it gives more pleasure than the vagina. Also, it feels different from the vaginal canal – not just tight, but smooth, offering them a different sensation."

Hurts so good?
From the female perspective, the physical sensation can be quite different – and painful! Why? "Most people have a muscle-contraction reaction in this area, to stop faecal matter escaping," explains Dr Angela Cooney, medical consultant for Family Planning Western Australia. "When you insert something into the sphincter, the muscle clamps down. You have to consciously relax to overcome that, which is difficult."

The solution is lube, and taking things slowly. The anus doesn't have a lot of natural moisture, so it's vital to use a

CHAPTER THREE

good quality, water-based lube. "Particularly the first time, insertion should be very slow," says Dr Morrissey. "Add lube as often as necessary. Breathe out as he inserts further, and talk it through as you go.

While the typical image of anal sex is for the man to position himself behind his partner, in a doggie style scenario, Dr Morrissey suggests trying out different moves. "The sitting position, with the woman on top, allows you more control," she says. "You can also do it in the missionary position or side-by-side." You need to be as calm as possible; if you're nervous, you'll literally constrict, making it more difficult. If it hurts, stop.

The hygiene factor freak-out

For many couples, pain isn't the barrier that prevents them from experimenting with anal sex. It's well ... poo. Though, according to Dr Cooney, there's not much chance of things getting messy. "The rectum is not a storage area for faeces; it's usually empty," she explains. "Faecal matter may be an issue if you're constipated or suffer from Irritable Bowel Syndrome," she adds, "but most people won't encounter anything untoward."

Good hygiene is vital when practicing anal eroticism. "Use condoms with anal sex, and use a fresh one to insert the penis into the vagina. You don't want to mess with the balance of bacteria in the anus and you certainly don't want to introduce bacteria found in the rectum into the vagina." Stay clean even if you're indulging in "hand play" in the anal area. "Wash fingers before and after inserting them into a rectum," Dr Morrissey advises.

THE MAIN EVENT

Don't underestimate the pleasure a man can receive through this kind of play. His G-spot is at the top of the rectum and it can give him a different kind of orgasm – streaming, instead of pulsing."

But is it dangerous?
So, can anal experimentation lead to any long-term health consequences? "Bottoms are not as robust as the vagina," says Dr Cooney. "Small tears and bleeding are more of an issue for penetrative sex in this area – and it's easier to transfer infections this way.

If you're in pain after anal sex, a cool water wash might help. "If you're really sore, look at your technique and ask yourself if it's worth it," she says.

If you practice anal sex regularly, there's another thing to be aware of. "Some people's sphincter muscles can become loose, leading to anal incontinence," warns Dr Morrissey. "But it takes decades to get to this point." It's more of an issue for people who like playing with oversized toys. Dr Cooney also says that long term problems are unlikely if you're "inserting something as relatively small as a penis" (I can hear men weeping the world over at this thought.)

Of course, you don't need to stop at a penis – sex toys designed specifically for anal eroticism are available. "If you're going to use toys, use ones that are specially designed," says Dr Morrissey.

CHAPTER THREE

Those hospital stories

So, is there any truth to those urban myths about people going to hospital in the middle of the night? "Small bottles and vases do disappear and have to be removed," says Dr Cooney.

"Toys should have some kind of stopper on them," offers Dr Morrissey. "If something disappears up there, you must go to hospital, which can be embarrassing, not to mention painful!"

Anal Sex Road Tests: Girls who've been there, done that

"I've tried it once - it bloody hurt. My boyfriend thinks I've opened the up-the-butt floodgates. I've told him the only time it'll happen again is on our wedding night."

Megan, 28

"I've never been into it, though I've tried it a couple of times, usually when I'm inebriated. And I tell you, it hurts like hell."

Louise, 26

"My ex-boyfriend was an anal freak; he was always at me to do it. I obliged a couple of times, but it just wasn't for me. I wouldn't say we broke up over it, but it was a factor."

Merryn, 25

"I almost did it once, but I was too anxious. The bottom line is this: it's bound to hurt and it could do damage. And it's poo, for God's sake!"

Kerry, 27

"You don't know what you're missing out on unless you try it. Once you get past the pain – which is only the first few times and is down to technique – it's the best feeling!"

Simone, 27

THE MAIN EVENT

THE A-Z OF SEX

Think you know everything? Hmm, maybe not.

Altocalciphilia: A fetish for high heels.

Basoexia: Arousal from kissing.

Candaulism: When two people have sex while another watches – often one member of a couple will watch his or her partner in the act.

Dogging: Stems from the idea of taking your dog for a walk in order to watch people having sex in cars. In known areas, couples leave the car light on as a sign that they are keen for an audience.

Erotomania: When a person develops an unreasonable love of a stranger or acquaintance who isn't interested in them.

Fluffer: The person responsible for getting porn stars aroused before their performance. Brothels also employ fluffers.

Gynonudomania: A compulsion to rip people's clothes off.

Hermaphrodite: A person who is born with both female and male genitalia.

Iconolagny: Arousal from pictures or statues of nude people and pornography.

Incubus: A mythological spirit thought to lie on top of women and have sex with them while they slept.

Jactitation: Becoming aroused by boasting about false sexual exploits to others.

CHAPTER THREE

Knismolagnia: Arousal from tickling.

Lectamia: Caressing in bed without coitus.

Merkin: A pubic wig that is often used by transsexuals or transgender people.

Naphephilia: Arousal from touching or being touched.

Odaxelagnia: Becoming aroused from biting another.

Pyrophilia: A sexual celebration involving burning. Sometimes chilli powder is rubbed onto nipples or genitals to induce a burning sensation. (Ouch!)

Queening: A form of domination where a woman sits on a man's head as if it were her throne.

Stigmatophilia: Arousal from a partner who is stigmatised, ie. has tattoos, piercings, scars.

Shrimping: Sucking someone's toes to turn them on.

Transvestite: Someone who dresses or acts in a manner typical of the opposite sex for emotional or sexual gratification.

Undinism: Arousal from water or having sex in a bath tub.

Vampirism: Consuming blood of partner for arousal. (Eww!)

Vanilla: The term for 'traditional', non-kinky sex.

Xenophilia: Becoming sexually excited by strangers, but once a seduction occurs, the thrill is immediately diminished.

Zelophilia: Being aroused by jealousy and the rush it provides. Zelophiles set up situations where their lover will solicit sexual attention from rivals.

THE MAIN EVENT

5 of the most overrated ways to get it on

1. **The Mile High Club:** You end up in one of those tiny, brutally lit, foul smelling toilets that more than 400 people have used in 3 hours. No thank you.

2. **Shower sex:** Cold tiles, water in your eyes and a slippery surface. Difficult to master as well as dangerous.

3. **Boozy sex:** You can't get your bloody bra off.

4. **Sex when you don't really want to but you're too tired to tell him to go home:** Always terribly quick (and terrible) and you'll hate yourself.

5. **Making your own sex video:** Deeply depressing. This makes the worst foreign film scene look like Hollywood.

A BONK A DAY KEEPS THE DOCTOR AWAY

Just because it's fun doesn't mean it's bad for you. In fact, say experts satisfying sex offers a mind-blowing menu of health benefits. Here are six medical reasons to do the wild thing.

1. It's a great work-out
Shagging takes energy, and the longer and more vigorous the bout, the more kilojoules you'll burn. A half hour session between the sheets consumes about 360kJ - that's a third

CHAPTER THREE

of a Mars bar (so if you ate the whole bar you better get busy!) Of course, lazy lovers lose less fat. So to maximise the benefits, adopt more active positions, such as you on top or standing against a wall. Straddling his thighs is certainly a more enjoyable way to tone thigh and buttock muscles than using taking the stationary bike for a spin.

2. It keeps the blues at bay
When you come, your body is flooded with neurochemicals, including mood-elevating endorphins and serotonin (which governs emotional states). Breast arousal stimulates the production of oxytocin, the "cuddle hormone". All three chemicals induce feelings of warmth and wellbeing. People who report having satisfying, regular sex are less likely to show signs of depression. I get happy just at the mere thought people might want to have sex with me.

3. It stops you from getting sick
A growing amount of evidence suggests that bonking boosts your immune system. Researchers of the University of Pennsylvania found that people who enjoyed frequent rolls in the hay produced nearly one-third more immunoglobulin-A antibodies than their less-active counterparts. And don't be selfish! Give, as well as receive, because studies show that offering pleasure can elevate your immune response for about three days.

4. It relieves headaches, stress and period pain.
Unless you've got a migraine, "Not tonight dear, I have a headache," is an illogical excuse to ditch sex. In fact, a romp might be the best thing for pain. It relaxes the body, distracts the mind and diverts blood flow from your brain to the surface of the skin. The same goes for period pain.

THE MAIN EVENT

Got cramps? Forget pills and pop an orgasm instead - it's a pleasurable antidote to those bellyaches.

5. It makes you look younger

A US survey by Dr David Weeks, co-author of *Secrets Of The Superyoung*, found that people who had sex at least four times a week looked younger than average - ten years (for women) and 12 (for men) - for their age. And it wasn't just the grins on their faces... Arousal and orgasm increase blood flow, improving circulation, oxygenating the skin and speeding up the removal of toxins. Add to that the fat-burning, muscle-toning benefits of a good sack-session, and it's hardly surprising that those of us who are getting more look better as a result of all the extracurricular exertion.

6. It increases your longevity

So, it makes sense that with all physical and mental benefits associated with a regular raunch, it's going to have a positive effect on life span. However, an extended diet of casual partners can shorten your life expectancy (as the single lifestyle has many risks associated with it). Now all you need is a mate...

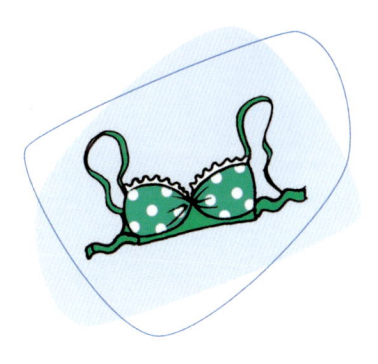

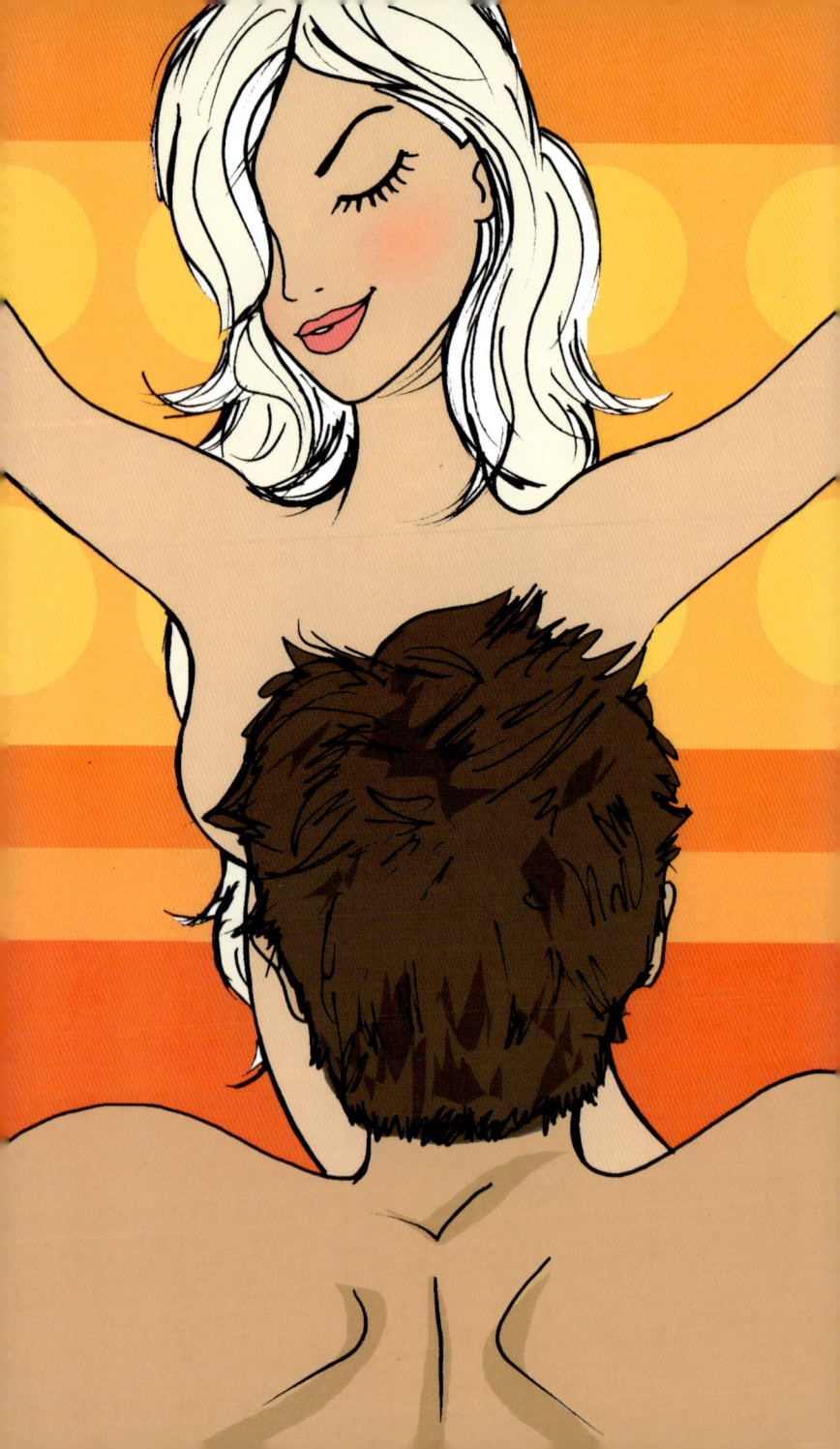

CHAPTER FOUR

'I'll have what she's having'

ORGASMS

CHAPTER FOUR

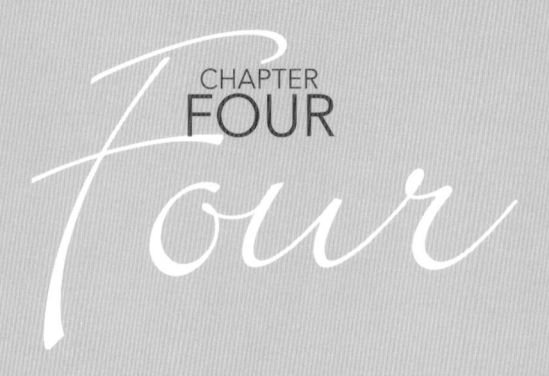

THERE IS ONE THING THAT SEPARATES A REGULAR SHAG FROM THE **OH-MY-GOD-DON'T-STOP** VARIETY. AN ORGASM. JUST THE WAY THE WORD SOUNDS, **O-R-G-A-S-M**, HINTS AT THE SCREAMING, SHUDDERING, CLUTCHING-THE-SHEETS SEX THAT'S SO GOOD YOU DON'T CARE IF YOU WAKE THE WHOLE STREET. I, OF COURSE, ENDLESSLY PANIC THAT I'LL WAKE THE KIDS, MY DOG - EVEN SOMETIMES MY HUSBAND - SO I HAVE JUST THE QUIET SHUDDERING KIND..

WHAT ARE THEY?

The physiology of an orgasm is best explained as a reflex action caused by sensation in the body. The stimulation can come from many sources but most commonly orgasm occurs after manipulation of the clitoris and sometimes the PC (pubococcygeus or pelvic floor) muscle as well. Although different stimulations may make the orgasm feel different, the physical reaction of the orgasm reflex is the same, characterized by rhythmic contractions of the PC muscle. That would be the shuddering bit I mentioned earlier!

ARE THERE DIFFERENT KINDS?

Most women distinguish between two types of orgasm. One result from direct clitoral stimulation, as in masturbation. This is characterized by a sensation more isolated in the pelvic area. The contractions of the PC (pubococcygeus or pelvic floor) muscle are more distinctly felt because the muscle is allowed to contract all the way since there is nothing inside the vagina.

An orgasm during intercourse differs in a number of ways, whether it is achieved through direct stimulation of the clitoris or not. The presence of a partner provides emotional charge which often heightens the response and women in studies have described how sensation takes over their entire body, briefly leaving her unaware of her partner or her surroundings. Feels good just writing about it!

Some experts also describe different types of orgasm - anal, nipple, fantasy, blended, etc - but these should give us enough to be getting on with it.

WHO'S HAVING THEM?

Well, facts are hazy on this one. A US study reported that 95 per cent of masturbation sessions result in orgasm (once you know what you are doing). During sex this figure plummets to 29 per cent for women and 75 per cent for men. Interestingly, 55 per cent of women said having an orgasm during lovemaking was not important to them (huge sigh of relief from male population). More bizarre statistics can be found on www.clitical.com (the site that "helps you hit the right spot"!).

CHAPTER FOUR

HOW ARE THEY HAVING THEM?

Time for a bit more snooping…

Do you have a sure-fire way to have an orgasm?

"I've never had an orgasm through intercourse alone. What turns me on most is having my breasts and nipples touched when I am having oral stimulation."

Jo, 31

"I mostly have orgasms through intercourse when I am on top and my clitoris is rubbing his pubic area. And I always have them during oral sex."

Lucy, 23.

"For the most explosive orgasms, I let myself go by taking deep breaths. This way I can build and control my orgasm yet still let it grow and explode all through my body."

Sandy, 29

"Sometimes I have sex in my lounge room while my flatmates are asleep upstairs. The thought of being caught adds to the excitement and makes my climax more intense."

Anna, 20

WHAT DOES YOUR ORGASM FEEL LIKE?

'My body shakes, I arch my neck and my thigh muscles tighten. Life is serene-for at least seven seconds, anyway!'

Angie, 19

I'LL HAVE WHAT SHE'S HAVING - ORGASMS

'A tingly feeling moves up from my knees until it arrives at my vagina. Then I feel several large contractions, followed by smaller ones. Sometimes it's possible to go on and have another climax. These feel different, beginning with an uncontrollable shaking, followed by a tingling sensation all the way up my legs.'

Nikki, 30

'Firstly, I have butterfly sensations in my pelvis. My clitoris is hard, my vagina and the muscles around the cervix tighten. My body is tense and I know I'm going to orgasm. The orgasm is quite violent but pleasurable. Afterwards, my heart beats very fast and there is a bright red rash on my neck and chest.'

Teresa, 21

WHEN IS ORGASM DIFFICULT FOR YOU?

'If I start thinking, 'Oh,no. I'm not going to come', or worry too much, then I don't come. I once had a boyfriend who used to ask me every five minutes if I was going to come - it put me totally off track.'

Eva, 22

'I need to be 100% in to what I'm doing. If I'm tired or have something on my mind it won't happen. I've never had an orgasm during penetrative sex so I masturbate.'

Janelle, 24

'Oral sex usually works for me, but not when I've been trying too hard or if I feel my partners heart isn't really in it. I get really annoyed when I can't come.'

Sandy, 21

CHAPTER FOUR

CAN I HAVE ONE?

Yes, you can.

As discussed in Chapter 1, masturbation is the best way to learn to climax. Becoming orgasmic isn't a matter of finding Mr Right. It's got far more to do with discovering what's right for you. Basically, successful sex, unlike piloting a light aircraft, is an activity that requires you to fly solo before you can take passengers along for the ride.

If you have trouble climaxing at all, even during masturbation, invest in a vibrator (see Chapter Seven) to help you find out what and where turns you on. If the sensations seem too intense, as they may do for beginners, muffle the vibes by putting a towel between you and your sex toy. However, enjoy the different sensations of a vibrator without relying on it for all your sexual stimulation. Otherwise you'll never leave the house.

Once you've mastered what pleases you, it's time to teach him. For most women this chapter isn't so much about having an orgasm as how to have an orgasm with a man.

Many women complain that when they have sex with a guy the earth doesn't move at all. Doesn't even twitch. He may be pressing all your buttons but he just doesn't seem to have your PIN number. There may be lots of reasons you haven't, as yet, climaxed with a man. Some of them may be to do with you, some may be to do with him (for instance if his idea of foreplay is unbuttoning his fly). Unfortunately, it's easy to get locked in to a negative sexual spiral. You didn't come. So next time, you're nervous. Desperate, even. Then, because you're uptight, the messages being transmitted

I'LL HAVE WHAT SHE'S HAVING - ORGASMS

from your clitoris to your brain, get hijacked by thoughts of expectation, doubt or the dishes still sitting in the sink.

The nearest equivalent in the opposite sex is impotence, with one crucial difference: for an impotent man there's no question of simply going along for the ride.

The Tingle Factor

Anne Hooper, author of *Sexopedia*, suggests this exercise in intimacy to help couples chart each other's ooh-zones:

- One partner sits nude in a comfortable chair while the other stands, then later kneels, in front. The object is to discover, through touching the body all over, which parts of it are sexually responsive.
- The partner doing the mapping strokes specific areas on his or her partner's skin, not more than 5 centimetres in diameter, once or twice with a finger.
- The person being touched rates the zones either high or low for eroticism. In this way you can build up a contour map of a partner's peaks and troughs of sensation
- This also chips away at any barriers between you (especially if you leave the lights on!). For women who have trouble coming, the better you know your partner - and he knows you - the better your chance of orgasmic success.

CHAPTER FOUR

WHAT'S STOPPING ME?

If you've never had one or are just having a dry spell it may be worth considering the following orgasm blockers.

Anger: You're mad as hell and you're not going to put out anymore.

I've never been a mad fan of "make up sex". If I'm pissed off I'd much prefer to be left alone to sulk. I'm quite fabulous at it and even if you've said your sorry it doesn't mean some "duvet dancing" is the logical conclusion.

While your mind may be saying "Nothings wrong. I'm fine", your body may be sending a very different message. "When a woman doesn't allow herself to admit anger, she may become sexually unresponsive," says Dr Harriet Lerner, author of *The Dance Of Anger*. "The body seeks the truth, and it's sending a signal that something isn't right."

But what can you do about this signal? Try putting on paper what you think might be the problem. Don't worry if the feelings seem irrational or unjustified: this is about how you feel, not about judging yourself. And once you know why you're upset, you can start dealing with it. If your anger is related to a specific incident (wet towels on the floor, him coming home at 3am or chatting up your best friend), talking about it might be enough. Bear in mind it may take two or three sessions for you to make your point and to let your anger rest. I know I can get pretty steamed up about wet towels on the floor.

Rule of thumb: pick a good time to talk. Forget a heart-to-heart over a rushed breakfast, straight after work or in a

I'LL HAVE WHAT SHE'S HAVING - ORGASMS

public place - even after sex is not ideal (as you may not hear yourself over the snoring). Instead, plan a quiet evening at home when there is less likely to be interruptions.

Says Dr Lerner, "Anger can certainly lead to intense sex but, in healthy relationships, your satisfaction in bed comes from love not anger." You will have an easier time making love to someone who doesn't make you furious all the time. Did you read that honey? NO WET TOWELS. EVER.

Poor body image: You think you're physically unattractive.

I have a mirrored built-in wardrobe in my bedroom. Useful when deciding what to wear. Less useful during daylight-sex. I can be happily in the throes of passion when I catch a side glimpse of the strange way my breasts flop to the side. I immediately transfer all my attention to my breasts. Why don't they sit up all perkily? Are those stretch marks on the side of them? Should I get a boob job? The passion is gone. He is going to pull a muscle before I ever manage to have an orgasm.

"Women have orgasms as a result of being comfortable with their size," says Catherine Lippincott, author of *Well Rounded: Eight Simple Steps For Changing Your Life... Not Your Size.* Nowhere is feeling comfortable with your body more important than in bed (except maybe at the beach lying next to my frighteningly perfect friend, Cindy). The good news is, if self-consciousness is preventing you from fully enjoying yourself there is a surprisingly simple cure: self-acceptance.

Truth is, we are often our own worst critics. Think about it. If you're able to forgive his love handles, why can't you accept

CHAPTER FOUR

them on yourself? It's time, girls, to give our other halves a touch more credit. Any decent man will accept you - lumps, bumps and all - because he cares for the whole package. Plus he probably hadn't even noticed your dimply bottom till you pointed it out. And don't forget, he has a hard on, is having sex, trying not to come too soon, trying to help you climax, his heart is beating very fast, there is blood pumping all over his body. Men aren't great multi-taskers at the best of times. Can you honestly say in the midst of all this, he is going to notice the odd dimple? Get real!

If you still aren't convinced, then invest in some beautiful lingerie, play music you love, light candles and engage your senses. If that doesn't work you can do what women all around the world do. Turn off the lights.

Mistrust: You don't trust him as far as you can throw him.
During her third date with Paul, Jane knew she was ready to take things further. So when he walked her home, she didn't hesitate to invite him in. They moved quickly from the couch to the bed and Jane was having a great time until he whispered, "You're the most beautiful women I've ever met. I think I love you." Eeek! Jane froze. "I realise some women would get off on that," she says, "but it seemed like a line to me. I don't need a guy to say he loves me to have good sex with him. But I do need to trust him. All of a sudden I started wondering, what am I doing? Who is this guy?" The pressure was on. All hopes of an orgasm were lost.

"Most women can't have orgasms unless they feel safe and comfortable and have a sense of trust." Says Sharyn Wolf, who wrote *How To Stay Lovers For Life*. If lack of trust in a new partner is coming between you and your orgasm, work out who your lover is and how you feel about him before you hop into bed. Having an orgasm is one of the most revealing things you can do in front of someone. If you can't trust him, trust your instincts and send him on his merry way.

Guilt: Your entire family is sitting on the end of your bed watching you.

Emily grew up in a strict religious family and was taught pre-marital sex was a sin. This belief didn't keep her from having sex before she was married, but it did make it impossible for her to enjoy it. "I first had sex when I was 19," she says. "My boyfriend worked really hard at trying to make me come but I felt like I was doing something so wrong that there was no way I was going to enjoy it. I loosened up with my second and third lovers, but I'm still dogged by guilt."

Even in these liberated times "sex is bad" messages are still common. Says Susan Quilliam, author of *A Woman's Complete Illustrated Guide To Sex*, "Women who have strong negative messages about sex, whether from religious teaching or a parent, often don't have orgasms because every time they go for it a recorder switches on in their brain that says, 'I shouldn't be doing this!'"

With a little effort on your part, the tape can be rewound and re-recorded.

Sharyn Wolf recommends a process called cognitive therapy, in which "old thinking" is replaced with "new thinking". The next time you hear your Mum's voice in your head saying, "Nice girl's don't" consciously and actively replace her words

CHAPTER FOUR

with some of your own. Tell yourself something like, "Part of being a healthy adult is having healthy orgasmic sex." Undoing decades of belief may take some time but if you persevere the voices will lessen and your sexual responses will get stronger.

The last (and very wise) point goes to a reformed friend of mine. She said, "Why on earth would God have given me a clitoris if he hadn't intended me to use it". Touché.

Stress:
You're too wired to even think about having an orgasm.

Last October, we bought our first home and between negotiating with mortgage lenders, packing up boxes, bubble-wrapping pictures, writing lists of my lists, I was also trying to work a full day as normal. Suddenly I had demands and deadlines. I'd wake up at 3am worrying if we could afford the mortgage or if I should have chosen oatmeal instead of cream for the kitchen cabinets (we settled on white gloss). In short, I was stressed. I realise that sex is potentially relaxing and, of course, it would have been - if only I'd managed to keep my mind on it. But every time my thoughts wandered off so did my orgasm.

"To have good sex," says Dr Lonnie Barbach, author of *50 Ways To Please Your Lover While You Please Yourself*. "You have to disconnect from the pressure of your environment and you can't do that when you are stressed. If you are somewhere else mentally, it's hardly going to work for you sexually either."

There are always going to be times when life is fuller or more demanding than usual but most of us get affected by day-to-day stress on a regular basis. So, how do you keep your mind on the game? The best strategy is to tune in to your body and focus on each physical sensation. Heighten these sensations by linking them to a visual image that turns you on - like a favourite position or erotic fantasy. Above all don't get stressed. Because getting stressed about how stressed you are is really stressful. Remember climaxing isn't the only way to have a good time, simple affection - kissing, hugging and squeezing - is satisfying in itself. And sometimes a good night's sleep is better than anything. You can always have an orgasm next time (be sure to remind him he owes you one!)

THE REST IS DOWN TO TECHNIQUE.

First things first: Foreplay. Yes please, lots of it; its value can't be underestimated. On average, it takes most women 45 minutes - yes, you read that right - from the beginning of sex until orgasm with a partner. Rely on penetration alone and you'll be sorely disappointed. So turn back to Chapter 2, which rants and raves about the benefits of foreplay and is highly recommended reading for both you and your lover.

THE POSITIONS MOST LIKELY

Fact: Some sexual positions are more likely to trigger orgasm than others.

For 29-year-old Karen, her orgasmic breakthrough "happened with a boyfriend who had a technique he called 'frigonometry'. Basically, it meant that he would deliberately rub his pubic area against mine - not too hard, not too soft - with every thrust. It was unbelievably wonderful."

CHAPTER FOUR

The problem with most sexual positions is that they simply don't make contact with the clitoris. Which as we all know is situated some distance from the vagina. Perhaps definitive proof that God is indeed a man. But the good news is there are positions which improve orgasmic odds such as:

Woman on top
Highly recommended for women who have difficulty reaching orgasm. This is provided you don't allow your man to move you around like a rag doll, but take charge and (if necessary) hold his arms down, as you work out the best way of gyrating over him.

Missionary position with a twist
You close your legs together and he puts his on the outside. He then raises his body and rests his weight on his elbows or outstretched arms. This places more weight on your pubic/clitoral area, giving lots of friction on the bits that count.

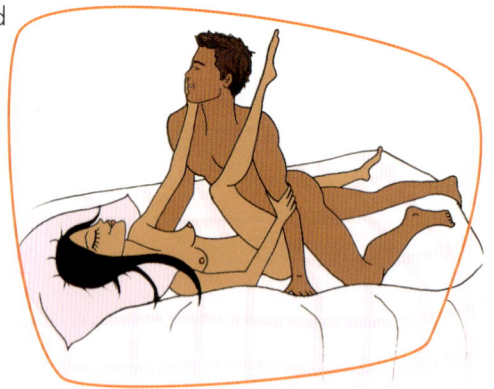

Doggy Style
This position allows for deep vaginal thrusting with the benefit that he can play a sonata on your clitoris at the same time ... this does rely on a degree of dexterity. Alternatively you can play with yourself. This is entirely within the rules of the game, since a very high percentage of women - more

I'LL HAVE WHAT SHE'S HAVING - ORGASMS

than 70 per cent - do not experience the "look no hands" variety of orgasm.

CAN I HAVE MORE THAN ONE?

Yes. A multiple orgasm, explains sex therapist Judith Seifer, is a "rippled" orgasm, which follows three of the four classic stages of sexual response - excitement, plateau and orgasm. The only difference is that instead of reaching the fourth state, resolution, the woman stays in the orgasmic stage, with peaks that are spaced about two minutes apart. If you do not have multiple orgasms, don't feel you're missing out: according to the website www.clitical.com, only 30 per cent of women have experienced multiple orgasm and just 10 per cent do regularly. Remember, quality is better than quantity.

WHAT DOES HE THINK ABOUT YOUR ORGASM

Question: How come it takes a woman so long to orgasm?
Answer: Who Cares!
Let's give the male race a little more credit than that. Here's what a selection of men really think it takes to get you there.

Is it important that your partner orgasms?

"Contrary to popular belief, most of the guys I hang out with do care about giving a woman an orgasm, otherwise they'd rather just masturbate. I have yet to meet these men that women talk about - the guy who roots and runs."

Chris, 32

CHAPTER FOUR

"Sure I do, it's a measure of my performance!"

Phil, 28

(Hmm... it's not all about you, Phil.)

"If the woman doesn't have an orgasm, you haven't had satisfying sex. For me, sex is very much an equal thing in that if a woman wants an orgasm and she doesn't get it, the sexual frustration is exactly the same. I think a woman should be just as forthright about what she wants and needs to be satisfied."

Rick, 27

How do you make sure she has an orgasm?

"Every woman is different. Some come directly from clitoral stimulation; some come when you put your fingers inside them."

Simon, 24

"Most women don't come through intercourse alone. These women are very fortunate. So I concentrate on positions where there is plenty of clitoral stimulation and pelvic contact. Like doggie style while playing with her clitoris."

Bill, 32

"It's all about anticipation and teasing - kissing her thighs, brushing her clitoris. You isolate the clitoris with one hand, spread the vaginal lips apart and softly tongue her whilst stimulating the inside of her vagina with your fingers. If you do that and then stop, kiss her thighs, then start again, you can build up a rhythm. Once you do that you know she's going to come."

David, 26

I'LL HAVE WHAT SHE'S HAVING - ORGASMS

What would you do if she couldn't have an orgasm?

"I'd raise the subject in a light-hearted way. You don't want her to think her orgasms are the be all and end all."

Gareth, 30

"It's never happened to me!"
(Sure, Dave, we believe you.) *David, 23*

"When it comes down to it, everyone's different and everyone attaches different things to sex. If emotions come into it and she's in love with you, her orgasm comes more easily."

Rupert, 29

Can you tell when a woman you're with fake's an orgasm?

"I can tell when a woman is faking it, but sometimes I'm wrong. A woman coming is a combination of many things. It's a shortness of breath in your ear, it's the trembling, it's the sudden stop. You become better at spotting a real versus a fake the longer you've been with a woman."

Charlie, 33

"It's easy for woman to fake orgasms. I bet I've been duped before without knowing it."

Doug, 25

"Absolutely. I can tell if she comes during oral sex, but during intercourse I can't tell. If you're stimulating the clitoris with your mouth and you have your fingers inside her you definitely know. The vagina expands and contracts - it swells up and then you have the contractions."

Brian, 30

(Quite the expert.)

CHAPTER FOUR

While we are on the subject...
FAKING IT.

I put this section last, because after all that precedes it, I hoped it would be null and void. But then I've faked it with the best of them so I can hardly berate you for having a quick peep. I think you would be hard pressed to find a woman who hasn't done the whole "Yeah baby" for his benefit. But there's little comfort in numbers: most of us have done it, but we don't feel good about it.

Any sexual put-on can leave you with misgivings and habitual faking can have serious consequences for a relationship. Although it often seems easier to pretend in the early stages, it isn't worth it in the long run. Your man will remember what it was he was doing at the time you rolled around in false ecstasy (rubbing, licking, stroking ... whatever). Then next time he'll be at it again (touching, fondling, nibbling), all for the sake of your pleasure. Which wasn't really pleasure to begin with. Nightmare.

A woman I know spent the first year of an otherwise promising romance faking most of her orgasms because she was too embarrassed to tell her boyfriend that his lovemaking style wasn't really hers. Finally, she found the courage to confess and suggested they experiment with some new techniques. They never did, however, because they never got back in bed. He was so thrown by the thought that her sexual climaxes were feigned that the romance sputtered and died.

In the end is faking an orgasm any worse than telling a lover the sex you just had was incredible when it was really only quite good? Or purring more loudly than necessary because

I'LL HAVE WHAT SHE'S HAVING - ORGASMS

you want him to know something he's doing is really working for you. I think we all have a little actress in us - and now and then it can be a useful talent. But mostly fibbing should be left for the more crucial things in life-like reducing the price of those fabulous new shoes you just had to have!

Female Ejaculation — IS IT A MYTH?

The issue of whether women can and do ejaculate is a tricky one. I have friends, both male and female, who swear that it is a reality. According to Lisa S. Lawless, author of *The Art Of Female Ejaculation*, it is a clear fluid, similar to prostate fluid. It is not urine and comes from the Paraurethral/Skenes glands and some women spray or gush out up to 2 cups worth! You can order her book and video from her website www.holisticwisdom.com and can even treat yourself to some graphic photos online. Yes, apparently, you too can soon be gushing...

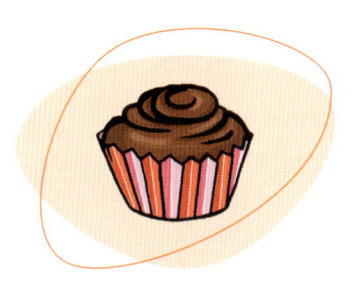

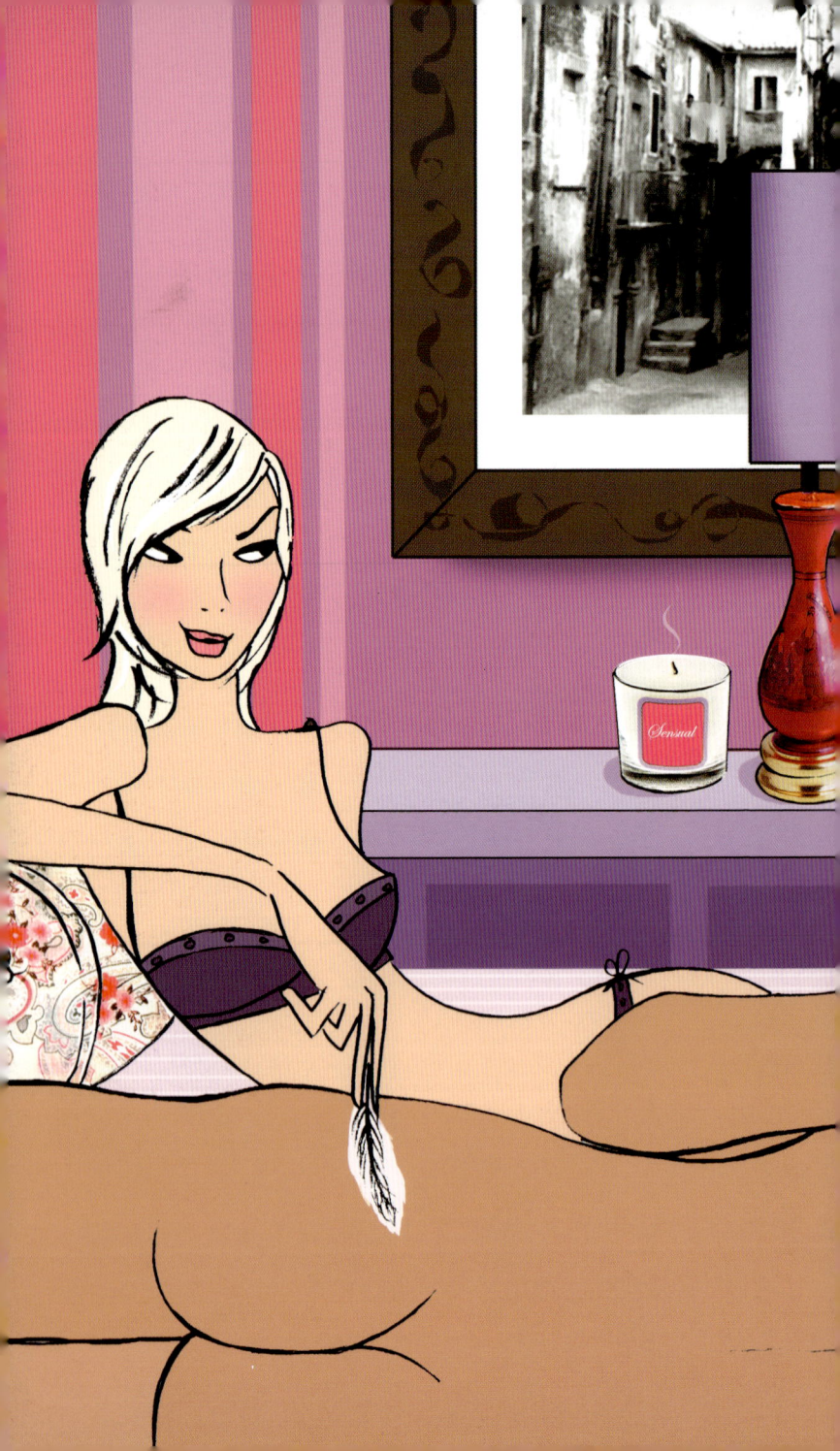

CHAPTER FIVE

Game Boy Advanced

WAYS TO DRIVE HIM WILD

CHAPTER FIVE

I ONCE RECEIVED A FABULOUS COMPLIMENT. WHILST IN FULL SEX GODDESS MODE WITH A NEW MAN, HE PULLED ME AWAY FROM HIM, HELD MY SHOULDERS VERY FIRMLY, LOOKED ME STRAIGHT IN THE EYE AND SAID, "YOU COULD BURN A MAN TO THE GROUND." SINCE THEN I HAVE MAINLY BEEN BURNING TOAST OR MY TONGUE WITH COFFEE THAT'S TOO HOT. BUT IN THAT MOMENT I WAS AT PEACE. I ALWAYS WANTED TO BE THE KIND OF GIRL THAT WAS 'GOOD IN BED'. AND HERE, FOR A MOMENT AT LEAST, I WAS.

I have just spent *weeks* asking men what makes a girl a great shag (fabulous opener at a dull party) and it can be summed up in one sentence: "If she's not too inhibited and enjoys herself. There's nothing better than a woman who loves sex." So lights on ladies, take the initiative and have fun! Can't be that hard really - can it? And lest we forget, the fact you are actually there and willing to have sex with him is half the battle. In the comforting words of my friend Mark, "I still can't believe women sleep with us to begin with. When they are lying there naked and smiling, it's like ... golf. It's like a championship round, when you hit an amazing shot that lands 10cm from the hole. If you make that putt, you

GAME BOY ADVANCED - WAYS TO DRIVE HIM WILD

win a million dollars. And you're praying you don't mess up. That's how I feel when I am about to have sex. I never know when I will get the opportunity again." I did mention to Mark that he may lessen his chances if he continues to compare everything to golf.

That said, the odd bit of technique doesn't go astray either. It's always reassuring to have a few tricks up your sleeve for a special occasion. So, we asked everyone from the experts to the boy next door, what a girl can do to raise her game to delicious diva level.

Ready to give him the ride of his life?

WHAT NOT TO DO:

Okay, let's get these out of the way first. Men are fairly straightforward when it comes to sex: if he's getting it; he's happy. So women can't go completely wrong. However, there are a few things that men request we do less of, or not at all.

- Lights off every time. Men are very visual creatures, let them look.
- Heading straight to Mr Happy. Believe it or not this shouldn't be the entire focus of the proceedings.
- Treating the male orgasm as a humorous spectacle.
- Ditching the sexy lingerie when you're in a long-term relationship.
- Always waiting for him to initiate.
- The starfish syndrome - where you simply lie on your back and let him go at it, as if sex with him is something you endure rather than enjoy.

CHAPTER FIVE

- Not giving him the verbal and physical feedback he needs to pleasure you better.
- Diving for his G-spot without checking he's receptive to the idea.
- Dashing to the bathroom as soon as it's over.
- Being embarrassed about your body. The last thing he's doing is evaluating your lumps and bumps.
- Falling into a routine where the identical foreplay pattern is followed every time by two or three positions that are always in the same order.
- Moaning someone else's name.
- Reacting to sperm as if it were sulphuric acid.
- Treating his penis like a pogo stick that's simply there to bounce up and down on, instead of a delicate instrument packed with nerve endings.
- Using your teeth on his penis.

A few other things that lessened the temperature were nagging, old-lady panties, body odour, pictures of your nanna by the bedside, etc. Hopefully things that by now you have eliminated all by yourself.

WHAT MEN WANT

Some things they want more of, some they want all the time and some they'd like to try at least once (pretty please). We asked what rocks their world.

"Bring me to the edge then stop, before doing it all again. It's like taking two sensual steps forward and one back, But, I know that when I finally climax, it will be incredible."

Trent, 32

GAME BOY ADVANCED - WAYS TO DRIVE HIM WILD

"Nothing gets me hornier than a woman undressing without saying anything. A girlfriend once stripped slowly in front of me while I was on the phone and I kept losing track of the conversation."

Jonathan, 25

"I don't like anything more than taking a hot drink to bed. Then I get my girlfriend to take a big sip of it, and when it's warmed her mouth she goes down on me for the best blow job ever."

Don, 29

"My ex used to flash parts of her body at me when we were out in public, like a nipple or a bit of inner thigh. It used to get me so horny. The delicious anticipation of it all."

Tony, 26

"I went out with a girl who introduced me to a great way of getting head. I put my penis on her tongue and, instead of closing her lips around it, she rolls her head in a circular motion, first clockwise, then anti clockwise till I am in heaven."

Peter, 32

"I enjoy coming between a woman's breasts, but even better is getting her to lie face down so that I rub my penis between her buttocks."

Josh, 25

"I used to love when my ex would spiral her tongue up and down the side of my torso. I wish more women would do it.'

Samuel, 30

CHAPTER FIVE

THE PENIS - A USERS GUIDE*
10 things to do with his penis you might not have thought of yet.

1. Holding it right. Not having a penis puts us women at a big disadvantage when it comes to knowing how to make one feel good. One of the biggest mistakes you can make is to assume what feels wonderful on your clitoris and in your vagina will feel equally wonderful on his genitals. Wrong. In case you hadn't noticed his penis is an altogether different animal. Whereas the general rule for clitorises is 'the gentler the better' for most penises it's 'the firmer the better'. So you should develop a grip for him something like the one you use on your tennis racket. But remember that you're dealing with a delicate instrument so don't crush it. The most sensitive area of the penis are the head, the rim at the bottom of the head, the long ridge running along the length of the underside, and probably the most sensitive spot, the slender string of skin connecting head to shaft on the underside (the frenulum). If you keep these hot spots in mind and use your fingers accordingly, you should have a happy penis in your hands.

2. Stroking it right. Now that your hand is strategically placed, it's time to get a little action going. Just three things to remember for the perfect stroke; do it firmly, do it smoothly and do it in a steady rhythm. If you want him to climax this way, increase your speed as he nears orgasm. But when he actually finishes climaxing, stop moving your hand. Either grasp him more tightly and just hold on or completely relax your grip and cradle his penis.

GAME BOY ADVANCED - WAYS TO DRIVE HIM WILD

3. Variations on the basic stroke: Knead his penis between both your hands as if it was a piece of dough (firm is good but too firm is painful).

4. Roll it between your palms but in this instance, like a cigar, keeping the "rolls" short and smooth.

5. Stroke the underside with your palm as you press his penis against your pelvis, steadily increasing speed and rhythm.

6. Press your breasts together and let him slide his well-oiled penis in and out between them. At the end of each stroke, let his penis emerge from your breasts and into your waiting mouth.

7. If your man has a high appreciation for women's bottoms, he will be sure to enjoy rubbing the length of his penis between the cheeks of your behind. Lubricate yourself there and present yourself from a kneeling position or lying on your stomach with pillows beneath your hips.

8. For an extra little treat, press on his G-spot whilst you are caressing his penis. The area between his anus and scrotum is called the perineum. Use your forefinger and press firmly and in rhythm while you stroke his penis with his other hand. If it's comfortable, you can curl the other fingers of your pressing hand around the organ base, using them to keep his penile skin taut. This sort of handiwork usually gives a longer-lasting orgasm (and top marks for you).

9. Whilst rubbing his penis cup his balls gently in your hand.

CHAPTER FIVE

Or, with thumb and forefinger on either side, press your fingers together between his testicles and pull down very gently as you stroke.

10. If you're bringing your man to climax by hand, you can simply loosen your pressure and stop pumping while he's actually in the throes of orgasm. Or you can try another method that may extend his orgasm briefly, try it and see how your man reacts. Keep up the stroking as he orgasms, but lightly. After he's ejaculated, confine your efforts to his scrotum and G-spot. Lightly pull on the shaft of the penis (stay away from the head) and massage his scrotum and perineum. This should feel to him as though you're hungry to "milk" him for even more juice and more contractions.

ORAL SEX

Yes, again. The man's enjoyment of this act can never be underestimated. We covered the basics of giving great head in Chapter 2 but there is always more to learn (and a willing recipient to practice on). Almost without exception, every man I asked admitted to trying to give himself a blowjob at some time. My friend Bruce even claims he had a rib removed! So we thought it best if we went straight to the top and asked men and women who give blowjobs in a professional capacity how to drive him crazy.

"Don't just go for the penis," says Sindy, who runs a massage parlour in Canberra. *"It's about working the whole area,*

(* From 203 Ways To Drive A Man Wild In Bed by Olivia St Claire. Copyright 1993 By Olivia St Claire. Reprinted with permission from Bantam Books Australia.)

GAME BOY ADVANCED - WAYS TO DRIVE HIM WILD

running your finger or tongue from his backside to the tip of his penis. It gives the guy the sensation of being really long. Take your time, tease him and if he's got foreskin, slide it around. Work the shaft with both hands, and then use one to play with his balls or perineum. Grab his balls with one hand, alternating heavy and light stroking. Then, using your tongue, work the head and the underside of his penis as if you're sucking on a lollipop. Make moaning noises while you're doing it. If the guy thinks you're enjoying it too then his pleasure doubles."

Selina, a fellow employee, recommends the stand-up blow job. *"It's a visual thing. Guys like to see their penis going in and out. Suction is more effective than trying to take his whole penis in your mouth,"* says Selina. *"But men get a huge kick out of this so, if you are going to give deep throat a go, use the sword swallower's trick of keeping your chin right up in line with your throat. If he's wearing a condom, keep going and pretend you're swallowing. Suck more gently after he's come and finish off with light stroking."*

Jarrod, who works for Global Male Escorts in Melbourne and knows a thing or two about what turns men on down under. *"Try using your hand like a cockring. Hold the penis right at the base really hard. Don't move. It just makes the rest of it really swell. If you can pull the penis out at a 90-degree angle it's in a position that his body's not used to. If you suck when it's in this position it's a lot more intense. The best way to deep throat is the 69 position. It's much easier because of the way the throats positioned. Breathe in through the mouth on your way down. You don't need to have your lips*

CHAPTER FIVE

around it when you go down, it's more when you are coming back up. And don't forget men are extremely visual. When the woman's down there and she looks up at you it's like ... Whoa!"

From my own personal "research", what works a treat is use the method above plus put both balls in your mouth and hum. You don't have to make any noise. It's about the vibration (which is a blessing, as I fail to hum in tune at the best of times!).

10 MORE WAYS TO MAKE A GROWN MAN SHIVER

Just in case you need something for a special occasion. Like the fact it's Friday or Saturday or Sunday... In fact, these tricks work just about any time.

1. Wear stilettos in the bedroom. It's a trademark of female porn and will make him feel like he's doing the deed with one of the centerfolds he masturbated over as a teen.
2. Dress up. In a nurse's uniform, two sizes too small. Give him a thorough examination, good seeing to and then tuck him in afterwards.
3. Drip candlewax on to his back. Just the ticket for men who like their pleasure with an aperitif of pain.
4. Pull at his pubic hair with your teeth, gently before you head for his package.
5. Pour champagne into his navel and chase the spillage with your tongue.
6. Go down on him when he is on a very important phone call with his boss or his mother.
7. Join him in the shower, with your PJ's still on - so he gets to peel it off before having his way with you.

GAME BOY ADVANCED - WAYS TO DRIVE HIM WILD

8. Meet him at a bar and pretend to pick him up.
9. During the day text message him all the things you are going to do to him that night.
10. Tell him during sex that you think he's "SO HOT, SO HARD, OHHHH, A MASTER LOVER, THE BEST I'VE EVER HAD." Or something along those lines. Must be done with straight face (a feat I have yet to master).

Drive Him Crazy — THE ULTIMATE EROTIC MASSAGE

The penis and scrotum: With your partner on his back, place a well-oiled or lubed hand over his penis and scrotum, fingers pointing towards the anus. Pull up toward the navel, sliding along the penis, alternating hands with each stroke.

The shaft: Cup one hand around the base of the penis and begin to slowly slide upward. When you reach the head, finishing the stroke with a twisting motion. Alternate with both hands in the same smooth motion.

Twister: Cup both hands around the penis and gently twist in opposite directions.

The anus: Lightly circle the rim of the anus.

Trust me - he will be completely at your mercy.

UNDERWEAR AND UNDER THERE

If you're expecting to get lucky it's worth giving a thought to the downstairs department. Despite the grand efforts you may have made in the fashion stakes, truth is most men don't really notice. Case in point, my man will tell me that "Danni looked really great last night." I'll ask what she was wearing

CHAPTER FIVE

and he'll have no idea whatsoever. Ask a girl and she'll tell you it was "Red top, no sleeves, black skirt - probably a Marc Jacobs - fishnets, black boots with a Cuban heel and a dangly pair of earrings."

That said, underwear and what lies beneath does get noticed because when you've got to that stage in the proceedings you have their undivided attention.

What he wants:

"I like very tiny, tiny G-strings especially in black or purple."
Sam, 34

(who probably also has a penchant for tiny, tiny bodies too!)

"Skimpy is good but texture is important. Stockings and suspenders are great and anything see-through goes down well."
Tim, 28

"I love when you catch a glimpse of a girl's bra peeping over the edge of her clothes. Very sexy."
Alex, 30

"You can't go past plain white undies. Especially if the girl is a lot less innocent than she looks."
Phil, 25

"If a girl is wearing really expensive lingerie, I know she takes care of herself. If I found out she had on a pair of old, greying knickers I'd be scared to go any further."
Vic, 28

"G-strings are overrated. Most girls just don't have the bum for them."
Mark, 30

GAME BOY ADVANCED - WAYS TO DRIVE HIM WILD

"There's nothing better than discovering she isn't wearing anything under her clothes."

Jim, 33

So be it a strip of lace, cotton briefs or going commando, make an effort - it will be much appreciated.

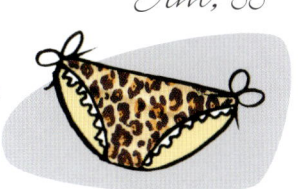

WHAT LIES BENEATH

A good wax is an easy way to boost your sexual confidence. I go a lovely lady who persuaded me to have my first Brazilian. She put it to me this way, "when a man goes scuba diving down there, he doesn't want to get seaweed in his mouth." Quite.

The Bare-All Details

What goes on during a Brazilian? Moving from the mound back, warm wax is applied, then removed, in small sections while you hold the skin taut. When a therapist reaches the more sensitive areas, the client's knees are bent to the chest, then rotated towards the shoulder as waxing nears the anus.

What He Thinks

"All that hair blocks the view, so I like some of it removed. You can see where you're going."

Colin, 24

CHAPTER FIVE

Beyond Brazil

If you want to go all out for a special occasion or you want to surprise him, some waxers will colour and shape your hair - hearts, lightning bolts and initials are all becoming popular. Expect to pay around $70 for a colour and shape. If this isn't really your thing, you may be reassured to know that in New York (where trends filter to our shores sooner or later), the bush is back. So whether you prefer a full head of hair, a landing strip or nothing at all, the choice is yours.

Sexual Pleasure:

"I get wet more quickly, partly because it's so sensitive but also because I feel sexier,"

Amy, 26

YOU WANT ME TO DO WHAT?!

A few of the really dirty things men wished you did in bed but are too scared to ask.

While satellite dishes can transmit messages to the far reaches of the universe, there's still an area - somewhere between a man and a woman - that remains something of a black hole. Men think about sex, talk about sex and fantasise about sex. What they don't do often enough is share their thoughts and desires with their partner - for fear of being labelled sexist, lazy, demanding, selfish or just plain weird. And so, in the interests of expanding sexual understanding between males and females, we got a guy to open up and tell us what men really want...

GAME BOY ADVANCED - WAYS TO DRIVE HIM WILD

Invite your best friend to join in.

This is assuming that your best friend is a woman, of course and, yes, we want to watch you have sex with her. What is it about lesbian sex that appeals so much, none of us can really put our, er, finger on. Men respond to visual stimulation, which makes us, by default, voyeurs. With two girls, we get twice the pleasure for the price.

Praise us.

On the odd occasion we are King Stud Muffin, tell us, "That was great." It's stupid, macho rubbish, we know, but we need it. Anything about the largeness of our penis also goes down extremely well. Conversely, when we are a bit off form, please avoid being too harsh.

Encourage us to have the odd quickie.

We spend a lot of our time trying not to come before you, so a quickie every now and then would be much appreciated. But do give us encouragement because that way, we don't feel so selfish.

Watch a porno.

We've been alone with our porn for far too long. It would be more of a turn on if you shared it with us. Please. It doesn't have to be full graphic, gynaecological guts and gonads material. Just something with a few bare bottoms and a bit of pants action. Look, laugh, and try out some of the positions and techniques. Then, if you feel like looking at something stronger, well, you only have to ask.

Bend over and show us your rude bits.

You may think your bits are funny looking. We don't. We love to look. Why not let us worship at the altar?

CHAPTER FIVE

Talk dirty.

It doesn't have to be a stream of profanities, just the odd rude word will do. It's even better if it's a rude word you don't normally use. "Fuck me hard, baby" is a good start. True, it's not romantic, but "I want to feel your wizzer in my tinky winky" doesn't really do it for us. (Does anybody really say that? If so, I hope they are reading closely).

Make lots of noise.

Moans and groans are not only sexy, they also provide an invaluable guide as to whether we are hitting the right spot at the right speed.

Let us have sex with your bottom.

We are not sure what psychologists would make of this one and, to be honest, we don't really care. What does concern us is how we can negotiate a tricky subject such as bottom sex. So in lieu of asking, you'll find men "accidentally" hitting the wrong spot. Anal sex is a bit subversive and we know we shouldn't be doing it. Which is exactly why we want to. Pretty, pretty please?

You have sex with our bottom.

We're a little shy when it comes to the subject of anal stimulation, with us on the receiving end this time, mainly because of its homosexual overtones. But the reality is, we'd really like you to tinker with our sphincter. The anus, say the textbooks, is blessed with a bundle of nerves that can cause a pleasant sensation when tickled, stroked or licked. Not too roughly, mind you. If I can say just one thing before you venture further afield: lubrication.

GAME BOY ADVANCED - WAYS TO DRIVE HIM WILD

Pleasure Probe

When it comes to exploring his butt there is a fine line between feeling captivated and feeling cavity searched. So do guys really like it? And what are the tricks to making that important little zone an erogenous one? We asked a selection of men for their top bottom tips:

"Be gentle, wherever you go."

"No sudden, jabbing movements."

"Keep your fingernails short."

"There's nothing like a tongue through the top of the bum cleavage, just before it starts to get in the crack. A lick through there, even if it's a flick of the tongue on the way up the back, is bliss."

"Butt cheeks must be caressed with both hands and kisses are an absolute necessity."

> REMEMBER: Always use a condom. Any kind of penetration, whether it's genital, digital or mechanical requires protection.

Masturbate in front of us.

We like to watch. We especially like to watch a woman masturbating and enjoying it. It is not only very intimate and sexy but, hey, we may even learn something.

Keep your knickers on.

We like underwear. Even better if there's a woman inside. So stripping off when you dive into bed is all very well, but leaving your knickers on is just as exciting. It gives us the opportunity to pull them off. We like doing that. Or even better, we can leave them on, pull them to one side and have sex with you while you're still wearing them. Very, very sexy.

Tell us what you want us to do.
While we aren't asking for a list of demands, the odd bout of dirty directives doesn't go amiss. This means you get what you want, when you want it - and we aren't left wondering if we should carry on with a few more hours of foreplay before we hop on to the fornication finale.

Tell us, in no uncertain terms, what you are going to do.
Anticipation is a fantastic stimulant, as is a running commentary of raunchiness. This works best if you whisper the saucy details in a conspiratorial tone, centimetres from our ears. Much better than sign language. Or telepathy.

Allow us a coffee break during cunnilingus.
It's enjoyable, believe us, but 20 minutes of tongue flicking and head shaking can cramp up even the sturdiest of sexual athletes. Serve cappuccino and biscuits and normal service will be resumed promptly.

OTHER THINGS MEN LIKE

I'm talking non-sexual stuff now. Most of these fall into two categories: Things That Can Be Consumed Easily, such as beer, pizza, hamburgers, take away, bourbon; and Things That Make More Noise Than They Should, which includes motorcycles, electric guitars, car horns. If you can incorporate any of his sexual likes into an evening that also includes items from the food and noise inventory - for example, a six-pack

GAME BOY ADVANCED - WAYS TO DRIVE HIM WILD

plus a monster truck show, or burgers and a rock concert - well, all I can say is, the man will be yours forever.

Burn a man to the ground? He'll be nothing but a pile of ashes.

My Favourite Fantasy — MEN TELL:

"Imagining my girlfriend sitting under my desk and giving me a blow job while I have a meeting with my boss. I have to try and keep a straight face as I'm having a mind-blowing orgasm and everyone talks business around me."

Leonardo, 35.

"Watching my wife have oral sex with another woman while I masturbate."

Joe, 26.

"Masturbating while a woman sits on my face. Just as she's about to come, she'd straddle me and we would explode together."

Andy, 27.

"Making love with a close female friend who I have always had the hots for. I'd like to tie her up and tease her until she begs me to enter her."

Graeme, 30.

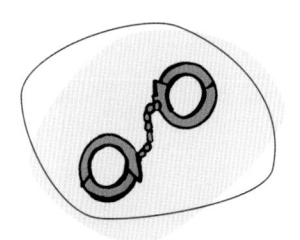

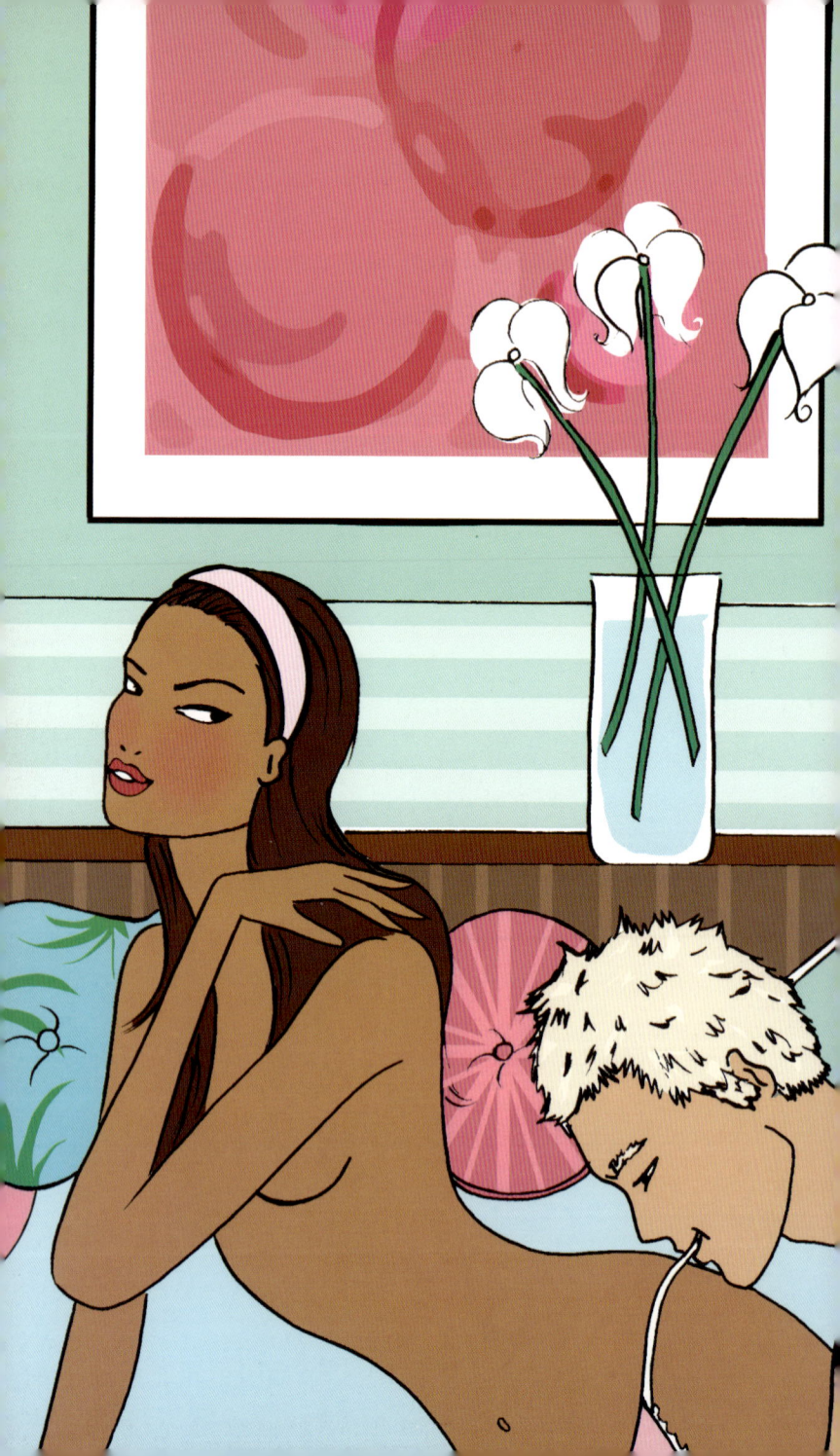

CHAPTER SIX

Light Her Fire

WAYS TO DRIVE HER WILD

CHAPTER SIX

AUTHOR ERICA JONG SAYS SHE KNOWS WHAT WOMEN REALLY WANT: "THE MAJORITY OF WOMEN SEEK A TRUCE BETWEEN THE SEXES, EQUITY FOR WOMEN WITHOUT SACRIFICING LOVE, AFFECTION AND EMPATHY. WE ALSO WANT HOT SEX, HARD COCKS, SURRENDER TO SENSUALITY AND, OH YES, ROMANCE."

What a complicated little bag of tricks women are! We want men to call, but not be too keen, to show affection publicly but not loose their masculinity, to bring us to the brink slowly and let us shudder to our conclusion - without noticing our thighs may be shuddering more than we'd like. The pressure to be all these things and more (not stingy, well dressed, clean, charming, confident, self deprecating, amusing, well hung) would bring most men to their knees (which ain't a bad starting position!). I must admit I sympathise. There's so much pressure for a man to know instinctively what we want and deliver it room service style. Without even getting a tip.

So if it's tips men need, they're on the right page. Leave this chapter open, girls, in a spot where he'll find it - like next to the beers or on top of the remote.

LIGHT HER FIRE: WAYS TO DRIVE HER WILD

WHAT NOT TO DO

Although we commend your enthusiasm when it comes to giving things a go in the boudoir, there are certain things best avoided if you want to be asked back.

Asking "Who's your daddy?" with a straight face. Ditto calling her "Mummy", which is likely to have her shooting out the door with her knickers barely pulled up.

Giving your penis a name that is cringe inducing. "Meet Russell the love muscle" is not a good look.

Even though most of us are fairly keen on receiving oral sex don't ask permission to "drink from the furry cup". Ali G may be funny but he's not a leg opener.

Both sexes I polled said that a tongue swishing around the insides of their ear is fairly repellent. Light nibbling or whispering is all that should be attempted.

Breasts: we know you love them but some of us are not that sensitive there. And please restrain from focusing on the nipples too much - all that squeezing, tweaking and biting can hurt.

The 69: it looks great in porn flicks but it's hard to concentrate on giving and receiving at the same time. It's sexier to take turns.

Never suggest a threesome on your first date. We'd like to think one of us is enough for you.

CHAPTER SIX

Asking us every five minutes, "Did you come? Did you come yet? Are you going to come?" We are trying, I promise, but you'll put us off our stride with all that pressure.

Jackhammer sex: where you just drill away at us till numbness takes over.

Taking yourself too seriously. Sex is funny. We are far more likely to have a good time if you relax and don't try too hard to be Super Stud between the sheets.

WHAT WOMEN WANT

Here's a few of her favorite things…

"I love it when my boyfriend ties me to the bedposts and works his way all over my body kissing, licking and stroking me. I never know where he is going to go next. The combination of pleasure and being helpless is such a turn on."

Kate, 29

"An ex-boyfriend used to suddenly assume a whole different character. He'd kiss me differently, touch me differently, say things unexpected, even his voice would change. Being taken by surprise was a real turn on."

Michelle, 30

"One guy used to have this move that would drive me crazy. He would turn me on to my stomach and blow gently and slowly down my spine, round the curve of my buttocks and tops of my thighs. Then he would raise my arse in the air and give me oral sex from behind. By the time he got there I'd be shaking so much I didn't care that the position was not that becoming."

Charlie, 26

LIGHT HER FIRE: WAYS TO DRIVE HER WILD

"Telling me what he's going to do just before he does it always gets me hot."

Sally, 22

"Never underestimate the power of a compliment. If you tell me I look sexy, I start to feel sexy."

Jana, 32

"I love it when a man lifts up my hair and kisses the back of my neck."

Lisa, 33

"It drives me crazy when a man gets his cock all oily and rubs it up and down my vagina before he enters me. This works particularly well with a Brazilian (wax or man!)"

Sam, 29

WHY DOESN'T SHE JUST TELL ME WHAT SHE WANTS?

We can hear your frustration. There are all these things we want and don't want and yet we sometimes leave you guessing. Flailing around blindly in the dark. Truth is we worry what you will think. Sometimes we just can't find the words. But if you listen closely you will tend to be able to hear better. If your finger is starting to head toward our bottom, and that's not our particular thing, we will squeeze our cheeks together or shift position. If you are going down on us, we might tilt our pelvis to try and get your tongue closer to our hot spot. If you are doing something good, we'll moan or arch our back or grab your arse. These are clear signals - just not in so many words.

CHAPTER SIX

A PLEASURE MAP TO
the Female Body

- Cover my stomach and breasts with chocolate sauce or whipped cream, then lick me clean. • Lightly run your finger or the tip of your penis from my neck and down through my breasts towards my vagina.
- Stroke my ego by telling me my tummy's sexy.

- Lightly stroke my fingers, wrists and the inside of my forearms. Use a finger or your tongue to make tiny circles in the palms of my hands.

- Massage my feet, ankles and calves with soothing essential oils. • Nibble, suck and blow on my toes.

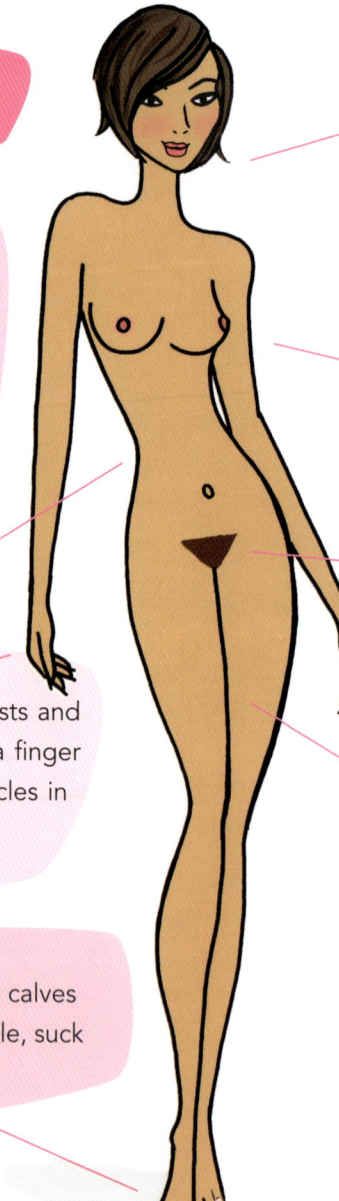

I'll have what she's having

LIGHT HER FIRE: WAYS TO DRIVE HER WILD

- Smother my, neck, shoulders, ears, eyelids, nose and lips with tender kisses.
- Gently rub the tip of your tongue down my neck, along my hairline and around my ears.
- Talk to me: whisper exactly what you're going to do.

- Wet my nipples with your kisses (or a piece of ice), then blow on them.
- Massage, nibble, suck and lick my erect nipples, but be careful not to bite.
- Gently hold my breasts together and stroke your erect penis between them.
- Tickle me-laughter is the best aphrodisiac.

- Tease and tantalise me by stroking my inner thighs.
- Slide your hand slowly up to my panties and feel me through the fabric.
- Remove my panties with your teeth or slide them off-slowly.
- Lick me gently, flicking your tongue over my clitoris. Cool your mouth with an ice cube for a tingling treat.

- Call my name when you come.
- Cuddle me when we've both come.

- Use a feather to lightly stroke my back, bottom, thighs and upper legs - don't forget the backs of my knees.
- Slather my stomach and thighs with oil, then slide your body slowly up between my legs.
- Tie me up with silken scarves and have your wicked way. But remember, it's only a game so don't spank me too hard and there's no need for all those Boy Scout knots.
- Grab the vibrator from my undies drawer and alternate gentle stroking (on low speed) with kissing and blowing.

CHAPTER SIX

Women like slow and gentle teasing. It's because we need a little more time to warm up and because the anticipation is what gets us really hot and ready. So after an evening of build up - talking us into a frenzy over dinner - take us home as dessert. Of course, just to be confusing, at times we want to be pushed down on the bed a little roughly and have our knickers ripped off.

THE FEMALE MAZE

A man's genitals are fairly self explanatory. They hang right out there for easy access and for all to see. Women, on the other hand, have most of their delights hidden and so it may at first feel rather confusing. Check out Chapter One for a detailed diagram.

CREATIVE TOUCHING

Women love it when men linger on different parts of her body. Diving straight for the genitals with a "Tally Ho!" and hoping for the best isn't the best approach. Erotic massage is a great way to warm up to a sexual encounter or the eroticism of the massage can be an end in itself. Whatever the preference, go slow and learn how to give and receive pleasure.

What he needs to know: Find a warm room, get her to lie on the bed and light some candles if you want extra brownie points. Go slowly over your lover's body so she can savour the sensations. Repeat each stroke up to a dozen times; be consistent, it's more soothing and relaxing. Ask what kind of pressure she likes, firm or soft, and adapt strokes accordingly.

LIGHT HER FIRE: WAYS TO DRIVE HER WILD

Erotic Massage techniques:

Full Body: Lay her face down, arms by her sides. Place a hand on each of her hands and travel lightly up the arms, around the shoulders and then down the body all the way to the toes. Without removing your hands, follow the same path back in the opposite direction. Repeat this stroke several times, adding more pressure. Then ask your partner to turn over and begin a scalp and face massage. Move on to the chest, arms, legs and feet. And finally the genitals.

Fanning: Place your palms face down side-by-side on her back. Simultaneously fan each hand out 90 degrees, then slide them gently up and down; bring hands back together and repeat the motion. The pressure should come from the heel of your hand or the thumb. Your fingers will feel wonderful grazing over the back, bottom, abdomen, thighs and chest.

Pulling: Place your hands next to each other on her side (fingers pointing toward the floor) and pull them up towards her spine or stomach if she's on her back, alternating hands. Or try it on the thighs, starting at the knees and moving away from the feet. Work up the inside of the thigh; the pulling motion tugs on the genitals, which can be quite arousing.

Massage toys and accessories

Feathers: Lightly run a feather over your partner's body for a sensation that even the lightest fingertips can't imitate. Long feathers are available from sex shops. Take care to avoid contact with body oil.

S&M gear: Whips and paddles can offer you a fabulous range of sensations, from a light slap to a hair raising sting. Bonds add an element of restraint to your massage.

CHAPTER SIX

Vibrators: They are often packaged as massagers so they may help. Experiment on the scalp, feet and neck and when you can't help yourself any longer, hone in on the genitals.

5 SURE FIRE WAYS TO REV UP HER SEX DRIVE

If all you've brought to the table thus far is a stiffy and some half-hearted clitoral stimulation, you're going to have to lift your game. There's only so long we'll be satisfied with no frills before we start wondering what gourmet tastes like. So if you're ready to release her inner nymph, add these devastatingly effective tactics to your repertoire and prepare to score.

A kiss before trying

Simple truth: women love to be kissed softly, almost hesitantly to begin with, then building up to slow, deep and wet. Why? Because it reinforces feelings of connection and the deeper this sense the more inclined she will be to get nasty. Kiss her like you've just met at a party, like the chances of taking her home that night rests on this one pash. Then repeat the process, letting things progress no further until, unable to resist your primal attraction any longer, she throws you to the floor/couch/bed and removes your pants. With her teeth.

Non-sexual touching

Unlike blokes, for whom being touched on the willy equals instant turn on, women can become aroused through contact that doesn't seem sexual in any way (we should in fact, come with instructions). Request she close her eyes, then trace her lips, cheekbones, eyebrows, eyelids and nose with your fingertips. Make like you're feeling the grain in seriously

LIGHT HER FIRE: WAYS TO DRIVE HER WILD

pricey timber. Listen carefully and you'll hear her breath rate pick up, she might arch her back towards you and she'll do a mental check that she's wearing sexy undies.

Get Necked
This is the part of her body so packed with nerve endings that even warm breath can tell the fun part in her pants to expect company. After spending at least 10 minutes pashing, slowly break away, brush her cheek with your lips and keep planting the lightest possible kisses on any skin your mouth comes in to contact with as you travel towards her neck. The key is softness. Imagine you're trying to lick a stray river of ice-cream that dropped on to your hand from the cone. No biting-large purple love bites are only for 15 year olds (who haven't worked out yet that they don't like them).

Breast is best
Tread lightly in this department. The way you treat her breasts gives many women a taste of how your performance might pan out downstairs. Gentle fingertips and warm palms are the ticket here. There is no need to head directly to the nipple. Explore the valley and tickle the seam between breast and ribcage with your tongue. Delay heading to the pointy bit as long as possible. When you do get there trace your tongue around the circumference, blow streams of warm air on to the nipple, then touch it with the tip of your tongue before eventually taking it into your mouth. (Mmmm...).

The Final Countdown
When heading downtown employ the same stalling tactics you did in nipple land. Run your fingers through her pubic hair, lightly drag nails over her inner thigh and plant feathery

CHAPTER SIX

kisses everywhere but 'there'. When you can't wait any longer (and she is begging you to go on) imagine you are at a fancy dinner party confronted by rows of cutlery. Stick to the rule of working your way from the outside in, and success is assured. Every woman responds to different things, but err on the side of tenderness and build from there as you see best. Finally, if you want to see her turbos flaming, experiment with different hand and mouth combinations until you find one that has her moaning thee loudest.

FOREPLAY FOUL-UPS

Where men tend to go wrong
(in a language they understand)

Penalty Offences:
- Touching yourself to hint you'd like her to pick up the pace.
- Pulling out of kisses when you want the "real action" to begin.
- Feverishly rubbing her crotch and nipples through her clothing. Friction burn plus nerve endings do not equal a turn on.

Yellow Card (10 minutes in the sin bin):
- Asking her to masturbate while you watch - lazy bastard.
- Placing her hand on Mr Happy before she is ready.
- Assuming that whispering obscenities in her ear will have her panting for it.

Red Card (You're outta here buddy!):
- Attempting penetration before she's ready (or awake yet).
- Twisting her nipples like you're turning a stubborn screw in to a wall.
- The dreaded head push towards the pants bulge.

LIGHT HER FIRE: WAYS TO DRIVE HER WILD

WHAT MEN WORRY ABOUT

Women spend a fair amount of time worrying if what they're doing is right. But what concerns does a man have?

Are women only interested in a big package?

Rest assured, women spend a lot less time worrying about the size of a man's penis than he does. Although not all men are created equal most men fall in to the "normal" range (between 12.9cm-14.9cm). Before all you men go fumbling for the tape measure, remember that a bigger cock does not equal better sex.

When it comes to sex, men can relax about the length, because he only needs a few centimeters for the job. The first 3cm of the vagina have all of the nerve endings and is most sensitive to stimulation. And if you believe it exists, the fabled G-spot is halfway up the inside wall. So you only need 4-6cm of penile penetration to rub her up the right way. A woman's vagina can accommodate most penises as it dilates even further when aroused. A bigger girth is sometimes preferred (ladies, a show of hands) as thicker penises are more likely to stimulate the clitoris during penetration.

It's also worth remembering that the biggest sexual organ is the brain. Being a good lover has nothing to do with the length of one's penis. It's about the lengths you'll go to satisfy her. So if you've got a tiny todger or a full-blown Tommy Lee, don't let size define your sex life. There's a whole lot more to it than that.

CHAPTER SIX

How to give good head

If your girlfriend doesn't seem too keen, it may be she's nervous of your reaction to the taste, smell and look of her. Reassure her and she is more likely to relax.

One Size Fits All

If he's big: Try it with him lying back and you on top. You can control the movement and depth of penetration. Lubricant will help too.

If he's small: Doggie style allows for deeper penetration with the additional option of clitoral stimulation. Another good one is spooning, with you in a foetal position and him entering from behind.

Women vary a lot in how they like their clitoral stimulation, some like it to be gently sucked, some can handle stronger flicking, some are so sensitive you can almost breathe in that direction and that's enough. Explore with your tongue, fingers and lips. "Vary what you do with your tongue. Author Harry Youngberry suggests you: "Use it pressed flat against her or edge deep in to her groove". Slowly retreat and lick your way back. Oral sex should be part of your foreplay and not just to get her to destination orgasm. However, if she is about to come when you are down there, don't change a thing - ride it out.

Grab a copy of *Mouth Music Made Easy* by W.D. Harry Youngberry. It's 68 little pages of how-to instruction. It will make you a very, very popular boy.

LIGHT HER FIRE: WAYS TO DRIVE HER WILD

How to give her an orgasm

Like men, women usually have their first orgasm on their own with their hands or a sex toy. Once women have learnt how, they'll try to have one with their partner. A few things hinder this: pressure, concern about how she looks and feeling confident and comfortable enough to let go. So, if it's not happening for her, it's not necessarily the guy's fault. It's something that both partners can work on.

Cunning Linguists

FIVE MEN AND THE TIPS OF THEIR TONGUES:

"Blowing gently on the labia for a minute before making contact has proved a winner for me."
Ben, 31

"My best tip is to pretend you are eating an artichoke. Slowly work your way from the outside in."
Angus, 24

"You can't beat a tongue that is flicking around like a garden hose on full blast."
Eric, 28

"A combination of mouth and fingertips always produces results. It's a two pronged attack."
Rowan, 23

"Sucking gently on her clitoris at the point of orgasm. But the key word is gently."
Mick, 30

I'll have what she's having

CHAPTER SIX

Communication (that old chestnut again) between two lovers is vital. She needs to show or say what turns her on; every woman is different but some things are universally true.

Longer foreplay is a good start. Lots of kissing, cuddling, stroking, teasing, licking, etc. Don't rush things and she'll find it a lot easier to climax. During intercourse, continue manual stimulation of her clitoris (or she can do it) as not many women can come through penetration alone. Some positions are better as they put pressure on the clit or the zinger G-spot.

Flip back to Chapter 4: The Main Event for position ideas. One posi that's top favourite is the pelvic slide: She lies on top and then, facing each other, get her to straighten her legs so they lie between yours. Then slide your body up and down, which will rub her clitoris against your pubic bone. Try this one tonight and she may even bring you breakfast in bed!

How to give her multiple orgasms

The shadow of the multiple orgasm looms over many a man's shoulder (I only gave her one orgasm - was that enough?) In truth, we are fairly happy with just the one but there is no harm in trying for more. Get hold of the book *How To Have An Orgasm ... As Often As You Want* by Rachel Swift. Read it together and then you can see what you need to do to help and how much she really needs to do herself.

The icky love stuff

Most women don't believe that love and sex are mutually exclusive. BUT (and it's a but worth mentioning) if she's in

LIGHT HER FIRE: WAYS TO DRIVE HER WILD

love with you then the sex can be hotter, more abandoned and more meaningful. I can't give you the magical formula that will guarantee she will fall in love with you (or I'd be writing that book in my vast waterfront mansion) but I can lead you in the right direction.

Tell her she is fabulous on a regular basis. Tell her how lucky you are. Tell her she is bright, beautiful and brilliant. And not just before you unzip your pants.

> "The basic conflict between men and women sexually is that men are like firemen. To us, sex is an emergency, no matter what we are doing we can be ready in two minutes. Women are like fire. They're very exciting, but the conditions have to be exactly right for it to occur."
>
> *Jerry Seinfeld*

Listen to her. Let her moan, chat, bitch and confide in you. Listen especially close to her in bed when she is telling you her wants and desires.

Show her affection in public. Women don't want to feel that you're embarrassed or ashamed to be with them. Just the occasional squeeze will do; sticking a tongue down her throat in the middle of the supermarket isn't necessary.

Don't suffocate her. Women want you to want them but not to the point that their life gets squashed in the process.

CHAPTER SIX

WOMEN TELL

My Favourite Fantasy

"Having sex in front of a crowd of strangers. They are not interacting but are just watching and getting aroused. I like to imagine them masturbating very quietly as they watch me make love to my partner."

Jodie, 32

"Being dominated by a man, and made to take off all my clothes, then having sex with another woman while he watches."

Carla, 27

"Making love with Brad Pitt and running my hands through his hair as he gives me oral sex."

Pip, 20

"Being brought to orgasm by my best friend (we're both straight), who shows me how to use a vibrator for the first time."

Angie, 23

"The thought of watching two beautiful strangers bonking each other senseless always turns me on."

Lynette, 28

"Having a threesome with my boyfriend and his best friend. I love the idea of having two men pleasure me. Funnily enough, my boyfriend's fantasy is having a threesome with me and my best friend!"

Helen, 21

LIGHT HER FIRE: WAYS TO DRIVE HER WILD

Turn her on. And wait for her to come. Women may take a little longer to join the table, but it doesn't mean they aren't as hungry as you are!

Stay for the after-party: Once the final orgasmic moan has bounced off the bedroom walls, this is not your cue to leave. For many women, this is where the real intimacy begins. Prolong her pleasure and she may even gear up for round two.

So what is it that women really want? It's not a big knob or even a big wallet (although a gift of diamonds and overseas travel was specified by my friend Sam). It's much the same thing you want (no, not a threesome): just someone who makes us happy, in and out of the bedroom. Do that and we will never leave you.

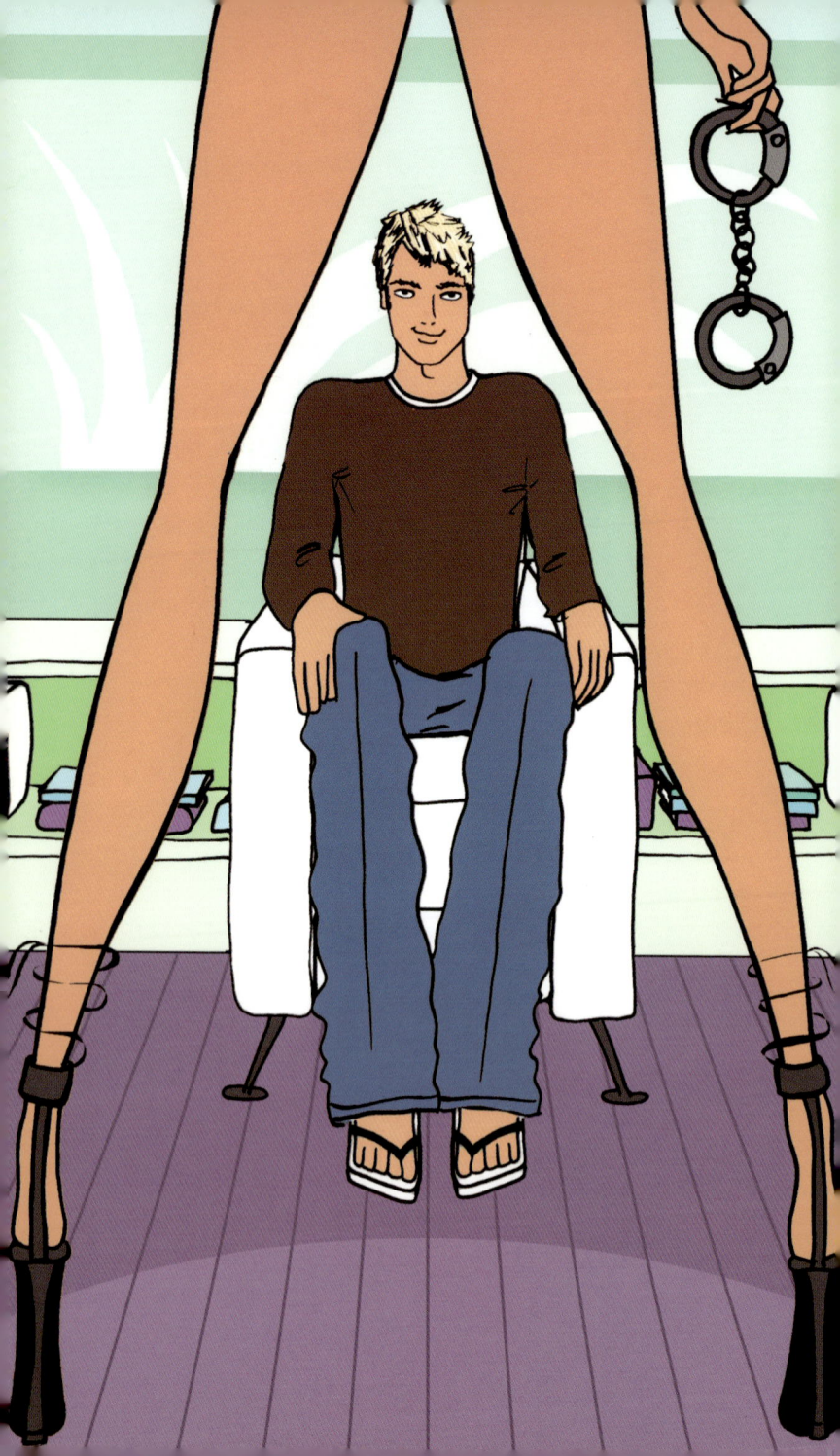

CHAPTER SEVEN

Batteries not included

TOYS, SERVICES AND OTHER STUFF

CHAPTER SEVEN

LIFE CAN BE A CRUEL, CRUEL THING. THE DAY I CAME HOME WITH A BAG BURSTING WITH SEX TOYS TO SAMPLE (STRICTLY FOR RESEARCH PURPOSES YOU UNDERSTAND - ANY ADDITIONAL PLEASURE WAS PURELY INCIDENTAL) MY HUSBAND SLIPPED A DISC. BEFORE I HAD EVEN UNWRAPPED THE FIRST LAYER OF TISSUE PAPER HE WAS ON HIS BACK YELLING LOUDLY. I HAD HOPED MY SUPPLIES WOULD HAVE THIS EFFECT, BUT NOT BEFORE I'D EVEN STARTED. HE SPENT A WEEK IN HOSPITAL SO I HAD TO TRY THEM INITIALLY ON MY OWN. WHICH, LETS FACE IT, ISN'T REALLY TOO TERRIBLE. BY THE TIME HE WAS DISCHARGED I HAD A PRETTY GOOD ANGLE ON ALL OF THEM AND WAS READY FOR MY SHOW AND TELL.

Before I started writing this book, I had one vibrator (the iVibe Rabbit - quite possibly the world's greatest invention), a few fiddly bits of lingerie and a French maid's outfit that I'd worn only once. I deemed myself rather paltry in the accessories department. I knew friends who had shelves of stuff; stuff to watch, stuff to wear, stuff that whizzed and whirled and made

BATTERIES NOT INCLUDED

them shout "Wahhhaay!" I've since discovered that for a few friends the cupboard is completely bare.

I took one of those friends with me on my shopping trip - she'd never been inside a sex shop (bless her), let alone asked for an in-store demonstration of each and every toy. She eventually left with a new friend tucked inside a brown paper bag and ducked home for an early night. The main thing I learnt that evening was that, behind the dark doorways and the neon lights, there is something for almost everyone. Even my friend, who left clutching her bag close to her chest, gave a quick wave and hopped on the No. 327 bus.

This chapter is all about accessorising your sex life. Whether you've been keen to try a piercing down there (brave girl) or just want to add to the toy cupboard, we've checked out all the extra things you can do, watch, try and buy.

GOOD VIBRATIONS:
YOUR LICK, TICKLE AND BUZZZZ GUIDE TO SEX TOYS

How to buy a sex toy

What are you going to use it for? If you're going solo and want to orgasm quickly, get a vibrator that stimulates the clitoris, or if you want to learn more about your body, go for something with some bells and whistles. Start with something simple. Opt for jelly or silicone toys, before moving on to the more high-tech stuff. Shop around - go on ask the assistant, don't be shy. Know where your clitoris and G-spot are, or you could end up with something that's too big or too long.

CHAPTER SEVEN

What should I buy?

Looking for the perfect buzz? Here's a few we tested.

VIBRATORS: They come in all shapes and sizes and are battery operated. The soft, squishy and flexible ones (made from jelly-like rubber, Cyberskin and silicone) are used internally; while the harder plastic styles are meant to be used externally. Some also stimulate both inside and out, as they come with a clitoral tickler.

First stop on my shopping spree was Miss Amour (114 Oxford Street, Paddington, NSW). This is a glamorous haven: all frilly lace, La Perla and tissue-wrapped sex toys. We asked the owner Sarah (funny, informative and totally unintimidating) for her hot sellers.

The Omega: This is their best seller. It comes in a racy red with stainless steel balls inside. It has seven speeds and seven pulses (that's 14 different ways to get a buzz on!). $199.00

The Pearl Rabbit: This is the one Charlotte in Sex And The City got her knickers in a knot over. A very reliable vibrator and sure to become a firm friend. $149.00

The Purple Rabbit: This is the best bet for beginners. It is smaller, less "cock-like", with no vein-like ridges. Popular with lesbians too. $139.00

The Hammer: This is quite something with front and back stimulators and unlike most, that go round and round, this has a back and forth action. $179.95

The Pleasure Ring: A vibrating, disposable cock ring that he puts on. It has a 20-minute lifespan, but Sarah assures me this gets the big nod of approval (this is from a lady who trials everything on an ongoing basis). She says it's like the perfect penis - it feels natural but vibrates perfectly for both your pleasures. $9.95

E-Glass Dildos: Made from Pyrex (it doesn't shatter). They look rather beautiful and you can heat them up or make them cold for different sensations. They are very hygienic because they can be boiled. They are smooth and slippery so easy to insert. Can work wonders on the G-spot. Oh, and you can stick them in the dishwasher. $120.00

Also in store, and now in my wardrobe, they have suede tasselled blindfolds and cuffs (bondage doesn't get any more glam than this!), feather ticklers and an array of costumes for the drama queens among us. No polyester in sight and most are under $100.

Next we ventured to the seedier side of the street and headed down the stairs to Club X (78 Darlinghurst Rd, Kings Cross, NSW). They have a vast array of toys (can I see a show of hands for the inflatable Pamela doll? Anyone?) and a video collection that would wear you out. Best tip they gave me is to check the speed variations on the tip of your nose, as it has the same amount of nerve endings as one's clitoris!

Here's a selection of other things you can buy:

The Tongue: A four-inch, naturalistic (for a giant) tongue with roughened surface and flexible tip. The tip wiggled like the real thing and as it comes with a power adaptor you can annoy your flatmate for much, much longer. You can position it between your legs and let it rip (or should that be lick). It's a little heavy for long sessions but in the hands of a well-built man it could be skillfully manipulated for maximum effect. $180. (I'd take the real thing over this any day of the week.)

Butterfly Clit Stimulator: A small butterfly-shaped vibrator (also available in dolphin and bumblebee shapes) with a harness that straps it onto your clitoris. Can be used during intercourse or around the house while you make dinner or watch TV. Surprisingly quiet, most models have multi speeds (worth checking). You can make the vibrations stronger by wearing underwear over top (helps hold it in place too). $44.95.

Love Balls: Hard, golf-shaped spheres that are attached by string. You insert them in to the vagina where they move around, creating waves of pleasure. Some women love them but many are put off by their size and it does make walking around a bit awkward. $19.95

Anal Beads: Four hard, marble-sized beads evenly spaced out on a string. You pull them out slowly of his anus when he climaxes. Men find the idea of this very exciting but it can be hard to time it right. $15.95.

Love Cuffs: Two pairs of nylon wrist and ankle cuffs with Velcro fastenings (safe alternative to handcuffs). If you feel safe with your partner and want to give yourself over to pleasure, these can be easier than rummaging around looking for a tie or a dressing gown cord. $12.95.

BATTERIES NOT INCLUDED

Erection Ring: This is an adjustable plastic ring that fits round the base of the penis to restrict blood flow, leading to prolonged erection. Guys get quite turned on by how hard and big they feel but it can become painful after a while and he might get freaked out if veins start to pop up. $14.95.

* If you're too shy to go into a store, log on to www.adultshop.com.au for discreet shopping that's delivered to your doorstep.

HOW TO INTRODUCE HIM TO YOUR SEX TOY

Mark, Meet Mr Good Vibes

In this age of post-feminist, post-HIV enlightenment, the humble vibrator has become many a girl's best friend. But telling that to your real-life sex partner is quite another matter. Still, with a little finesse and forethought, you can have him enjoying the sex-toy experience as much as you do. Here's how to do it, without damaging your reputation or his ego:

1. Don't threaten his masculinity by introducing a XXL-sized dildo. Start with something that's small and cute. The less it looks like a penis, the better.
2. Make sure it's quiet. There's nothing like the sound of a two-stroke motor to turn a shy guy off.
3. Let him watch you do it, then ask him to take over because your hand's tired. Tell him it's twice as much fun when he helps.
4. Reassure him that there are things he can do that a sex toy will never be able to do – such as kissing your breasts, licking your inner thighs or murmuring sexy words in your ear.

CHAPTER SEVEN

5. Turn the vibrator off occasionally, grab his (hopefully swollen) member and moan, "Gotta have the real thing!"
6. Definitely don't groan long and loudly a minute after starting up your sex toy.
7. Try your mechanical mate out on him – in a pain-free, playful manner. He might be as fond of the feeling as you are (in my humble experience, he will be).

What the boys said

This is how four red-blooded males responded to the issue:

"My girlfriend came across an ad for vibrators at the back of a magazine. She said casually, 'That's disgusting', but I could tell from the tone in her voice that she didn't think it was disgusting at all. We started talking about it and, the next thing I know, we're in a sex shop stocking up."

John, 35

"If she was the one to introduce a sex toy, it'd be all right – as long as she didn't pull out something bigger than mine!"

Richard, 25

"I've never had a relationship where we didn't eventually experiment with sex toys, so I don't have any problem with it. Why not try something new?"

Andrew, 33

"I had to go away for six weeks for work and my girlfriend informed me she would have to unleash her trusty vibrator in my absence. I told her she'd have to let me in on the action when I got back."

Alex, 28

BATTERIES NOT INCLUDED

Switched On

Worried that your electric dreams could turn into a nightmare? Here, we answer your most frequently asked questions about sex toys.

Q "My boyfriend wants me to use my vibrator on him. Does that mean he's gay or bisexual?"

A In a word, no. Sexual preference has nothing to do with how you like to be stimulated. I suspect you may be alluding to whether he wants you to use the vibe in anal play – again, this does not imply anything about his sexual preference. Many people find the skin around the anus highly erogenous. Relax, let him guide you and have fun.

Q "Can vibrators be dangerous? For instance, can I electrocute myself?"

A It really depends – if you're using an electric massager, it carries all the risks of any battery-operated device, so take all the usual precautions and certainly don't use it near water! I haven't heard of anyone being zapped by a vibrator but, nevertheless, if you read the instructions, some do say "Not for internal use". Do remember to take the batteries out when not in use, because they can leak a toxic fluid.

Q "Can continuous use of a vibrator damage the nerve endings of my clitoris or vagina? Is it possible that I could be permanently desensitised?"

A Nerves can certainly be overloaded by stimulation, which can reduce their sensitivity for a while. However, by the same token, women often complain that their clitoris becomes hypersensitive when it's over-stimulated. I think you'd have to be using your vibrator an awful lot to cause any damage. In fact, you'd need to be buzzing away all day and night and, even then, the batteries would probably give out before your nerves did!

Q "I've never had an orgasm. Could experimenting with sex toys be the answer?"

A Women who have difficulty achieving orgasm often also say they don't masturbate. The issue is not whether you should use sex toys but whether masturbation will help you, and I think it will. The key to orgasm is being comfortable with your body and letting yourself go with the flow to find your pathway to orgasm. This is why being alone, without any pressure to perform, may help. A good first option is those little vibrating butterflies; they provide consistent stimulation to the clitoris without the intimidation of a dildo.

PORN

I was hard pushed to find a man who didn't have a penchant for porn, even if some of them no longer indulged. Part of the appeal is that pornography is a retreat from responsibility, a ride to instant gratification where the pleasure is all theirs with no need for opening doors, meaningful chats, contraceptive preambles and stray pubic hairs. It is a fantasyland, an adult Disneyland, where you don't have to queue for a ride.

Women on the other hand, found it harder to balance their feminist principles with pages of naked girls with inflated assets and insatiable appetites. But I spoke to a lot who were as keen as men.

BATTERIES NOT INCLUDED

What she thinks

"For me, porn is almost like a fantasy that I wish I could act out. You know, not to be ashamed of my sexuality, to be completely free to take on as many guys and/or girls as you please and just f%#* till you feel content."
Louise, 25

"I was very upset when I discovered my boyfriend's video collection. I didn't want to be a prude but I didn't want him buying into Playboy's definition of sexuality because I was never going to look like one of those girls."
Jennifer, 28

"I read lots of erotica. I like it better than visual porn. The brain is the biggest sex organ and my imagination is very vivid. I also read all sorts of magazines of this genre to get turned on or just tune out from everyday life."
Maxine, 29

What he thinks:

"I watch porn with my girlfriend, on my own and even with mates over a few beers. It's got to the point where nothing shocks me anymore."
Sean, 32

"Reading a magazine and having a wank is much easier than seducing a real woman."
Jim, 21

"My girlfriend and I really get off on watching dirty movies together, especially the girl on girl action."
Jim, 27

"I don't know any man who isn't interested in watching women with no clothes on."
Stan, 21

CHAPTER SEVEN

"Porn is a big part of my life, but I don't really tell anyone. My wife would kill me if she found out."

Steve, 33

"I get hundreds of e mails a week from mates, each more filthy than the next. Most are more amusing than a turn on."

Ted, 29

VIDEOS

Did You Know?

According to the Eros Foundation in Australia, the average age of a woman watching her first X-rated video is 22; of those surveyed, 57 per cent were in a live-in relationship.

My trip to Club X taught me that there is a video for every kind of fetish you might have; from the rather extreme, "Arse me no questions: Anal road trips" to the more soft-focus, female-friendly "Vivid Collection".

Many sex shops will allow you to exchange your videos, saving you 50 per cent on your next purchase (useful for those that are keen to have a revolving door of porn into their homes). Downloading films from the Internet is the lazy girl's way to get off.

Recommended viewing (especially for first-timers): Anything by Jenna Jameson; something from the "Vivid Collection" or "Wicked Collection" - these movies are aimed at the female market.

How-to videos: These may suit your sensibilities more and you can learn a few things at the same time.

BATTERIES NOT INCLUDED

KAMASUTRA ($30) Each position is road tested by actors, but the demonstrations of the most difficult positions require more explanation. Especially for those without a gymnastic background.

LOVERS GUIDE 1 ($39.95) This aims to show couples in long-term relationships how to stimulate each other and keep sex interesting. Quite matter-of-fact but good close up shots of female genitalia, which show what happens when you are aroused.

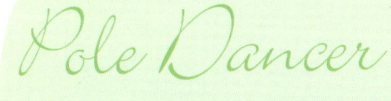

Pole Dancer

If you are looking for a novel way to get fit, have some fun with friends and delight your man why don't you try pole dancing?

Polestars: They run six-week courses for $200 in Sydney, Melbourne and Brisbane. Log on to www.polestars.com.au

Bobbi's Pole Studio: Located in Sydney and Perth, it runs specialty classes like lap dancing and exotic dancing. For more info: www.bobbispolestudio.com.au

Pole Divas: Take an eight-week course or casual classes in Melbourne. More info at www. poledivas.com.au

EROTICA

Did You Know?
According to the Eros Foundation, Aussies purchase 1.5 million sexually-explicit magazines and books each month.

CHAPTER SEVEN

Many women prefer a good story to get their imagination going. Recommended reading alone or out loud with a partner:

Unruly Appetites: Erotic Stories by Hanne Blank (Seal Press, $27.95) Twenty Erotic tales to titillate, intrigue and inspire.

Naked Erotica edited by Alison Taylor (Pretty Things Press, $14.95) Twenty-six stories of naked lust.

Sweet Life: Erotic Fantasies For Couples by Violet Blue (Cleis Press, $27.95) Explicit stories of couples who try out their No. 1 sexual fantasies.

CYBERPORN

Did You Know?
Sex is the most requested subject on the web.

There is very little you can't see on your computer in the comfort of your own home. There is a global peep show on the World Wide Web and nobody is more than a click away from "Hard Core Action". Luckily, pornography that tunes into what women really want is a growing market.

Recommended sites:

www.forthegirls.com For a site that's raining men and that boasts "kissing, cunnilingus and afterglow" - stuff that's usually left out of mainstream sites.

www.couplespleasuredome.com A site where you can download female friendly DVDs with helpful sectioning of categories such as Fantasy, Intimacy and Storylines.

www.sssh.com An online magazine with pictures, stories, advice and discreet shopping.

BATTERIES NOT INCLUDED

PIERCING

A whole universe of piercing exists beyond the ear lobe. And for those of you brave enough to go there it's all about pain before pleasure. Dr Richard Janus, Australia's top piercing expert and founder of www.bodyartdoctor.com tells us everything we need to know.

"A piercing will only enhance pre-existing sexual response," says Dr Janus. A piercing won't automatically make you orgasmic. Learn to use the basic equipment before seeking an upgrade!

The who, what and where

Horizontal clitoral-hood: This piercing, usually a ring, passes horizontally through the hood of the clitoris. Healing takes three to five months but you can have gentle sex a few weeks after the piercing. In contrast to the vertical hood, this piercing doesn't provide direct clitoral stimulation. Instead it can be pushed onto the glans clitoris or tugged and played with in a partner's mouth during sex.

Vertical clitoral-hood: This piercing passes vertically through the clitoral hood, and rests at the head of the clitoris itself. Known as the "walking orgasm", 75 per cent of women with this type of piercing will experience increased pleasure during sex. And a small number will climax when they least expect to. Like, in the supermarket.

Guiche: Location wise, this is a rare choice. It goes through the skin between the vagina and the anus. Have the entry and exit points shown to you in a mirror before going ahead and discuss jewellery type and positioning. Six-nine months

CHAPTER SEVEN

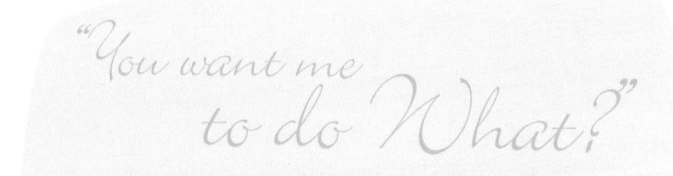

"You want me to do What?"

SEX WORKERS SPILL THEIR WEIRDEST REQUESTS:

"A guy once asked me if he could put his fingers down my throat and make me throw up a little bit on him. Only problem was, once I got started, I couldn't stop and ended up repeatedly vomiting on him."

Mandy, 24

"One of the funniest clients I've ever had didn't even want to have sex, he just wanted someone to play fairies with him. He'd arrive, change into a tutu, ballet slippers and wings and we'd spend an hour throwing glitter around and dancing to music."

Greta, 24

"I was asked to act like a cat. I thought the client must have had a fetish for Catwoman but it turned out he was sexually attracted to his neighbor's cat. So I had to miaow, crawl around, pee in the kitty litter and wear a fur coat."

Cassy, 25

BATTERIES NOT INCLUDED

healing. As it is very complex only allow a master piercer to do the work.

Minor Labial: This describes any piercing of the labia minora. Discuss at length the jewellery size and position with your piercer. You can resume intercourse (gently) within a few weeks.

Genital piercing and sex

Intercourse: Some enjoy the extra sensation, while others may find it too intense. Many piercings can be taken out (or put in) for lovemaking.

Health Alert: Until any genital piercing is healed you have an open wound and a portal for diseases into the body. Practice safe sex and don't forget saliva can transport disease too.

How do I find a good piercer?

Log on to www.safepiercing.org – its members meet strict criteria.

Source information on websites such as www.bodyartdoctor.com and talk to people who have already been pierced.

Ask questions: Is their equipment sterilised? May you see it? If they won't show you, assume it doesn't exist and leave.

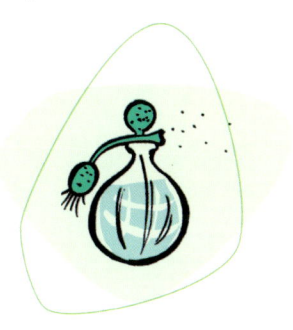

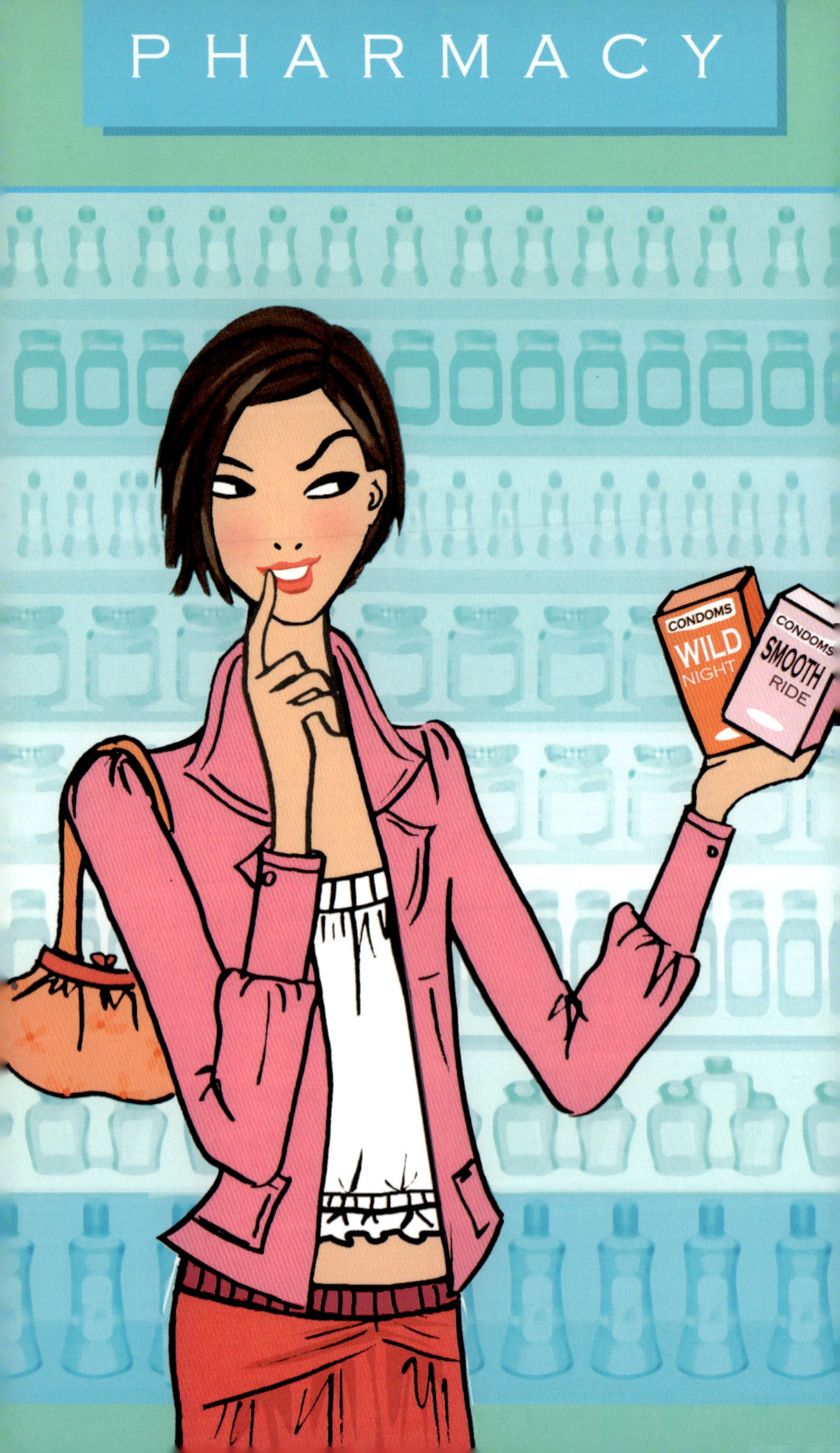
PHARMACY
CONDOMS
WILD
NIGHT
CONDOMS
SMOOTH
RIDE

CHAPTER EIGHT

'Protect your assets'

SAFE SEX

CHAPTER EIGHT

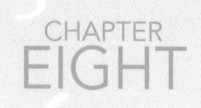

THE ONLY REAL WAY TO HAVE COMPLETELY SAFE SEX IS NOT TO HAVE ANY AT ALL. NOT MANY OF YOU WOULD BE TICKING THAT BOX. SO, THIS CHAPTER WILL BE LOOKING AT THE VARIED WAYS TO MAKE YOU SAFE, NOT SORRY AND PROTECT YOUR ASSETS WITH MINIMUM FUSS.

Back in the '80s the Grim Reaper advertising campaign saturated prime time TV. The message was stark. AIDS is here and it can kill you. For a while, the scare tactic worked. For the majority of people in the '80s and '90s, safe sex became a routine. If you had sex, you used a condom.

Fast forward to Noughties and it seems we all are suffering from safe-sex fatigue. The 2004 Global Sex Survey from Durex reveals 54 per cent of Aussies had sex without a condom. It's time to get savvy about the facts regarding STIs (sexually transmitted infections).

SAFETY CHECK

What can you catch from a guy through sex?
Many things, ranging from relatively harmless to seriously damaging viruses, some of the potentially fatal. According

PROTECT YOUR ASSETS

to staff doctors at the Melbourne Sexual Health Centre, the most widespread viral problems they see in men are genital herpes and genital warts; both are highly contagious in their active phases. Of the bacterial diseases, the most common in Aussie males is non-gonococcal or non-specific urethritis (NSU), usually contracted via a female sex partner who has Chlamydia - an often symptomless condition, thus easy to pass on.

How do you know you have an STI?

Sometimes you'll have symptoms: vaginal discharge; soreness or itching; cold sores or small warty growths on your vulva. But, at other times you won't notice anything. The common, but dangerous, STI Chlamydia - a virus transmitted to girls from guys with NSU (and back again) - can be symptomless in both sexes. The best way to ensure you're clean is to see your doctor, sexual-health centre or family planning clinic. Check ups at specialist institutions, including those at public hospitals are a good option - they are usually free. See our STI chart for a more detailed look.

What are the signs he might have a STI?

It's no simple matter. Some STIs have no visible symptoms, and, even if he's aware he has an infection, he may not tell you-especially if he thinks it might scare you away. So, it's a good idea to check him out. Keep the lights on and, during foreplay, have a good look (and feel). Don't be shy – but be careful with your hands, as certain infections are contagious during skin-to-skin contact.

If he has any reddish, possibly weeping sores (or small, flat scabs indicating them) on or near his genitals, perineum or

CHAPTER EIGHT

anal area, it's possible he has herpes. Run your fingers over his genital and anal area and check for cauliflower-warty lumps or little flaps of skin: these could be genital warts. If you squeeze the glands of his penis and a discharge emerges that looks cheesy and/or creamy, rather than the clear pre-ejaculatory fluid, it could be a sign of gonorrhoea or NSU. None of which sounds like the kind of foreplay to get you revved up!

There is no way of telling if he's HIV-positive, short of asking him – and he may not know anyway. Ditto with syphilis. So a girl's best defence against STIs is the good old condom, and carefully conducted foreplay.

What's the best way to bring up the issue of STIs?

Soon, and straightforwardly. There's no point beating about the proverbial bush here, because if you're bonking a guy you aren't in a monogamous relationship with, you must insist he wear a rubber.

What do you do if you think you have an STI?

Tell him - and any other sexual partners you've had prior to identifying the infection.

What do you do if you find out you have had prior to identifying the infection. Say you're sorry to be the bearer of bad news, but you figure it's better to let him know up-front than him to find out further down the track, by which time he might have unwittingly infected others. Remember there's also a possibility he gave you the problem in the first place. Pass on to him the number of his nearest sexual-health clinic too - if you make it simple for him to get treated, he's more likely to do so.

PROTECT YOUR ASSETS

So, how do you treat STIs?

Don't ever attempt to self-diagnose or treat STDs - unless you're a chronic thrush sufferer and you are sure that's what you have. These days STI scans are simple, free, confidential and painless. If you're sexually active and not practicing monogamy, it's smart to have an annual check-up with your Pap smear. Fortunately, most common infections are now treatable with creams, pessaries, cold-laser application or antibiotics.

STI ALERT: What Every Woman Needs To Know

Get smart and protect yourself with this must-read guide to sexually transmitted infections.

CHLAMYDIA

What Is It? A bacterial infection of genitals or anus.
How Many People Have It? 20,026 reported cases in 2001.
How Is It Transmitted? During vaginal or anal sex.
Symptoms: Vaginal discharge; pain during sex or when urinating; abdominal pain; bleeding after sex and in between periods. But 70 per cent of women have no symptoms. It is detected by a swab from the cervix or anus, or a urine sample.
Treatment: Antibiotics - a single dose or a ten-day course.
If Left Untreated: Pelvic inflammatory disease (when the reproductive organs in the pelvis become inflamed). PID can cause ectopic pregnancy (when pregnancy develops in the fallopian tubes instead of the uterus), pelvic pain or infertility.

CHAPTER EIGHT

GENITAL WARTS

What Is It? Caused by the Human Papilloma Virus (HPV).

How Many People Have It? More than 30 per cent of the population is believed to be infected.

How Is It Transmitted? During sex and direct contact with an infected person's skin.

Symptoms: Usually appear three to 18 months after contact. They include itching; inflammation; warts or cauliflower-like clusters in the genital or anal area. Detected by the appearance of warts or by a Pap smear.

Treatment: Warts can be removed by freezing, laser or surgery. But even with treatment, recurrences are common, as there is no cure for the virus.

If Left Untreated: Some variations of HPV have been linked to cervical cancer.

GONORRHOEA

What Is It? A bacterial infection of the genitals, anus or throat.

How Many People Have It? 6,158 reported cases in 2001.

How Is It Transmitted? During vaginal, anal or oral sex

Symptoms: Appear two to ten days after infection. Yellow or greenish vaginal discharge; a burning sensation when passing urine. But two out of three women have no symptoms. Detected with a swab from the cervix, anus or throat, or a urine sample.

Treatment: Antibiotics.

If Left Untreated: Pelvic inflammatory disease, ectopic pregnancy, infertility.

PROTECT YOUR ASSETS

HEPATITIS B

What Is It? A virus that causes infection in the liver.

How Many People Have It? 424 reported cases last year

How Is It Transmitted? Sharing needles and syringes, contact with infected blood, sex with an infected person or an infected mother can transmit it to her new baby.

Symptoms: Appear four weeks to six months after transmission but there may be none. Flu-like symptoms; loss of appetite; night sweats; whites of the eyes go yellow; fever; pain in joints; nausea; vomiting. Infection is detected by blood tests and liver damage is detected by a liver ultrasound.

Treatment: Not necessary unless liver damage occurs. Then antiviral injections or tablets.

If Left Untreated: 95 per cent of people get rid of the virus and then have lasting immunity. About 5 per cent retain the virus and may be at risk of cirrhosis and liver cancer.

HERPES

What Is It? Caused by the herpes simplex Virus (HSV). HSV-Type 1 causes facial infections such as cold sores and can cause genital infection via oral sex. HSV-Type 2 causes genital infection. Approximately one in eight Australians carries the virus that causes genital herpes.

How Many People Have It? Approximately one in eight

How Is It Transmitted? Through sex with a person carrying the herpes virus. It invades the body, often through a crack in the skin or via mucus in the mouth or genital area. It can be transmitted during oral sex given by someone who has a cold sore.

CHAPTER EIGHT

Symptoms: Tingling, itching, burning or pain, followed by the appearance of painful red spots that evolve within a day or two into whitish-yellow fluid-filled blisters. But in many cases, there are no symptoms. Women often experience pain when urinating. Diagnosis is confirmed by a physical examination and a swab from a blister or genital secretion during a suspected herpes episode.

Treatment: Antiviral tablets. Can be taken each time you have an outbreak or daily to suppress outbreaks occurring. Salt baths to keep the area clean. Visit your local GP or sexual health clinic to get The Facts Pack now, or check the website: www.thefacts.com.au

If Left Untreated: Outbreaks recur but it is not life-threatening and doesn't affect fertility.

HIV

What Is It? Human Immunodeficiency Virus (HIV) affects the white blood cells and destroys the body's natural ability to fight infections. AIDS (Acquired Immune Deficiency Syndrome) is a group of illnesses that result from the weakened immune system in people with HIV.

How Many People Have It? There are about 450 people newly infected each year in Australia.

How Is It Transmitted? Can be sexually transmitted via anal or vaginal sex without a condom.

Symptoms: Doctors can test for infection with a blood test three to six months after contact. In the early stages, HIV can trigger flu-like symptoms and a rash. Later symptoms may be swollen glands, diarrhoea, night sweats, fatigue, minor oral and skin conditions.

PROTECT YOUR ASSETS

Treatment: There is no cure, but the disease can now be managed. Antiviral treatments reduce the amount of HIV in the body, and side effects can include diarrhoea and nausea. A large number of tablets need to be taken every day. It is important not to miss a dose, to ensure that treatment works.

If Left Untreated: Eventually HIV weakens the body and makes it vulnerable to serious infections. This stage is what is referred to as having AIDS. There is no cure for it but people with AIDS can live for many years.

CONDOM CONUNDRUM? NO WAY.

As discussed condoms are the ONLY way forward until you are in a monogamous relationship and you are both declared 'clean and clear'. After which time, there is a whole different world of choice out there. Trial and error is sometimes the best way to proceed. I've been on various pills, on and off over the years and some make me horny (fab), some make me grumpy ("Not in the mood. Don't even think about it.") and some have made my cleavage larger

Q. How do you put a condom on an uncircumcised penis? All the instructional pictures I've seen only show circumcised ones.

A. A lot of sex education material is visually old-fashioned. Even though most men before 1970 grew up without foreskin, the current national circumcision rate is between 10-20 per cent. However putting on a condom is exactly the same whether the penis is circumcised or not; when fully erect, the foreskin of an uncircumcised penis naturally retracts.

CHAPTER EIGHT

(extra fab) but also most of the rest of me larger too (no fair!). So, whatever your concerns or requirements, here are all the answers to start you on your way.

CHOOSING A CONTRACEPTION

It's a Fact: There will never be a 100 per cent, one-size-fits-all contraception method that caters perfectly to your sex life. It's just a matter of finding one that suits your body and your lifestyle. Read our chart and then consult your doctor to find the best one for you. It's important to remember that this is just a guide and not all women have the same experience with the same method of contraception.

THE COMBINED PILL

What Is It? Also known as "the Pill", it's an oral contraceptive containing the hormones oestrogen and progestogen, which combined stop you from ovulating.

How It Works: You take one pill a day in a 21-day or a 28-day cycle, have seven days off, then start the cycle again. There are many types containing different levels of hormones.

Suitable For: It's suitable for most women, but some may experience side effects due to the hormone levels and may need to try a few brands before finding a suitable one.

Unsuitable For: Women who find it hard to take a pill regularly. There's a greater risk of pregnancy if a pill is missed or taken 12 hours later than usual.

Possible Side Effects: Nausea, breast tenderness, spotting and mood changes.

Effective: 97 to 99 per cent

PROTECT YOUR ASSETS

THE MINI PILL

What Is It? The mini pill only contains progestogen as opposed to the oestrogen/progestogen in the combined pill.

How It Works: It makes the mucus of the cervix thicker so sperm can't get through to meet an egg. The 28-day cycle of pills should be taken at about the same time each day.

Suitable For: Women who experience nausea, high blood pressure, weight gain or headaches from the oestrogen in the combined pill.

Unsuitable For: Women who have irregular periods and a history of ovarian cysts.

Possible Side Effects: Prolonged periods, heavier periods, irregular periods, or no periods at all and spotting.

Effective: 96 to 99 per cent

LONG-ACTING HORMONAL INJECTION

What Is It? An injection that contains a long-acting hormonal contraception called medroxyprogesterone. Similar to the pill. It stops you from ovulating.

How It Works: It is given to you every 12 weeks by a doctor or nurse and will work immediately to prevent pregnancy if started within five days of your period.

Suitable For: Women who can't use contraception containing oestrogen, have difficulty remembering to take oral contraceptives or who find other methods unreliable.

Unsuitable For: Women who've been menstruating for only

three years; suffer depression; have high-blood pressure; a blood-clotting disorder, or irregular periods; are diabetic.
Possible Side Effects: Headaches, weight gain, irregular periods and loss of libido. There may also be a delay in fertility once you sto the injections.
Effective: 99 per cent

FEMALE CONDOM

What Is It? The female condom is a polyurethane sheath about 15cm long and is pre-coated with lubricant.
How It Works: With two flexible rings to hold it in place, it forms a loose lining in the vagina and acts as a barrier to semen and other bodily fluids.
Suitable For: Women who don't like to use hormonal contraception, people who have an allergy to latex and partners who find it hard to maintain an erection with a condom on.
Unsuitable For: Men and women who need lots of lubrication. It can also be difficult to insert and does take practice to do it properly.
Possible Side Effects: None are known.
Effective: 95 per cent

THE COPPER IUD

What Is It? The intra-uterine device (IUD) is made of flexible plastic with a fine copper wire wound firmly round it. It's toxic to sperm and prevents the fertilisation of eggs.
How It Works: Placed in the uterus; has nylon string for easy

PROTECT YOUR ASSETS

removal. It should be checked six weeks after insertion and then every year thereafter. Replace every five years.

Suitable For: Women who don't want more kids but want a long-term yet reversible form of contraception. If pregnancy occurs while using the IUD, it must be removed.

Unsuitable For: Women who have heavy periods; have uterine abnormalities; have never had kids; or are at a long-term risk of contracting STIs should not have an IUD fitted.

Possible Side Effects: Increase of bleeding, painful periods and vaginal discharge; risk of infection after insertion. IUD may expel itself during a period, unbeknownst to the user.

Effective: 99 per cent

DIAPHRAGM

What Is It? The diaphragm is a dome-shaped rubber cap worn in the vagina during sex.

How It Works: Fits inside the vagina and covers the cervix, acting as a barrier to stop sperm entering the uterus. Remove at least six hours after intercourse, as sperm can live for hours.

Suitable For: Women who only want to use contraception when required, or need to find an alternative to hormonal contraception.

Unsuitable For: Women who suffer vaginal infections, or have vaginal or uterine abnormalities, as the diaphragm may trigger more problems.

Possible Side Effects: Increased risk of urinary tract infections and discomfort to the vagina due to irritation from the diaphragm's latex coating.

Effective: 84 to 90 per cent

CHAPTER EIGHT

HORMONE ROD

What Is It? A small rod containing the hormone progestogen; it's inserted under the skin of the upper arm under local anaesthetic.

How It Works: It steadily releases small amounts of progestogen into the body to prevent ovulation. Lasts for three years and can be removed at any time by a GP.

Suitable For: Women who have difficulty with remembering to take oral contraceptives or with using other methods. Suitable for suffers of oestrogen side-effects.

Unsuitable For: Women who experience irregular bleeding, take medication (as it may affect the implant) or who don't like the idea of an implant under the skin.

Possible Side Effects: Weight gain, acne, headaches, breast tenderness and changes to periods.

Effective: 99 per cent

REAL PEOPLE, REAL STORIES

We didn't use condoms, now I've got two kids.

Vicki, 19, is a mother of two sons, aged 17 months and four months. Her first son's arrival was unplanned and the result of unprotected sex.

"I'd been with Matt for seven months when I fell pregnant. When we started having sex, we never used condoms but I was on the Pill. Matt didn't want to wear them - he said they were uncomfortable, and I went along with that. I think it's hard to get a guy to wear a condom if he doesn't want to.

PROTECT YOUR ASSETS

We weren't planning on starting a family at such a young age. At the time I fell pregnant, I'd had a bout of food poisoning and was given medication to treat it. I didn't realise but somehow the medication made the Pill less effective. I was about to turn 17 when I found out I was pregnant and it was a huge shock. I asked Matt what he wanted to do and he said he wanted to keep the baby and stay with me.

I went to the GP to confirm the pregnancy and immediately the doctor said 'Okay, we'll organise a termination before it's too late.' Because I was young, there was an automatic assumption I'd want an abortion but personally I don't believe in it.

I was working in a bookshop at the time but I lost my job because the owners were quite religious and said they weren't comfortable with my situation i.e. that I was young, pregnant and unmarried. The pregnancy wasn't easy. I've had moments when I've wondered how we'd cope and I lost friends because they didn't understand what I had to deal with.

Once my first child arrived, Matt and I decided we wanted a second baby fairly soon so that the kids could grow up together.

We use condoms now - we don't want more children and we realise how easy it can be to fall pregnant. You need to think, if you don't use a condom, would you be able to look after a child?

Recently while I was in a supermarket, I saw a woman look at me with my children and then tell her daughter, 'Don't you

CHAPTER EIGHT

dare end up like that'. I've been called a 'slut' and a 'baby-making machine' because I'm young and a mum. Maybe we could have done things differently, but I could never be without my children now. I think any woman who is having sex needs to stop and think about her life and remember how quickly it could change if she doesn't use a condom."

Herpes: It happened to me

Christy (name had been changed), 28, a customer service officer, was devastated when she was diagnosed with herpes four years ago.

"One of my best friends in high school caught herpes the first time she had sex. I was revolted and automatically assumed she must be a bed hopper. I was 17 and thought only dirty girls got STIs. I had a boyfriend and I remember thinking, 'She'll want to sleep with him now.' I assumed anyone with something so awful couldn't have any morals. Now I realise how naïve and wrong I was.

I first had sex with that same boyfriend when I was 19. When we broke up, it took me a few years to get over the relationship. I dated a few other guys and, at 23, met the man I thought was The One. Until then, I'd always insisted on using condoms. I was brought up in a strict religious household that didn't believe in sex before marriage. The fear of falling pregnant and my friend's experience with herpes kept me practicing safe sex. But a year after I started dating my new partner, we stopped using a condom. It seemed like a natural progression.

A few months later, I felt really sick at work, as if I had the flu but without the sore throat and blocked nose. The following day I didn't feel any better. During my break I sat on some steps outside to get some fresh air and realised I could feel only one bum cheek. I had a strange tingling sensation in the other.

After what happened to my friend at high school, I read up that flu-like symptoms and tingling were typical of herpes. I just knew I had it. My instincts told me. The following morning I went to a sexual health clinic - I couldn't go to my doctor because I was so embarrassed and ashamed. A nurse found a herpes rash on my genitals. It looked nothing like a cold sore. It was actually so tiny I couldn't see it.

When I told my boyfriend, he immediately asked who else I had slept with. I'd been 100 per cent faithful, but he said he couldn't possibly have infected me and refused to get tested. He also told me he didn't need a girlfriend with problems and dumped me.

I don't know whether he was the person who infected me - I might have had herpes for some time and not noticed - but I was devastated when he left. In a couple of days my life changed completely. One day I had everything, the next I had a disease I'd never get rid of and no boyfriend. I felt I could never trust anybody again.

For the next few weeks I couldn't stop thinking about it. I was terrified people would look at me and know I had herpes. To make up for it, I went to the gym religiously and was always immaculately dressed. Two weeks after the diagnosis, I almost had a breakdown because of the shock. I didn't think anyone would love me again. Then my sister pointed out

CHAPTER EIGHT

that, if a guy runs when you tell him you have something as simple as a cold sore, then he's not worth it.

I started taking anti-viral treatment when I was diagnosed and I've taken medication on and off since then. I've been on anti-viral medication to suppress the virus for the past 12 months because I'm in a stable relationship. I've had other outbreaks but they've not been as severe as the first episode. I know when the virus is active - I get a funny sensation in my leg, like the feeling of being sunburnt. When that happens, my partner and I don't have penetrative sex. The rest of the time we use condoms and dental dams.

I told my partner I had herpes the first night we met. He just asked if he could take me out for dinner the next night. He read about herpes and we both know what we have to do to minimise transmission. It's never easy to tell a partner, but if a guy likes you he won't reject you because of it.

Herpes has been a wake-up call for me. You think these things only happen to 'dirty' people and that you'll be able to spot the guy with the STI - he'll be the one with bad jeans and hair - but you don't know. Herpes is a reminder that I'm lucky, I could easily have been infected by something much worse."

Helpline
For more information on sexual health, go to
www.fpahealth.org.au *or* **www.thefacts.com.au**

PROTECT YOUR ASSETS

Don't think that these things only happen to other people. It could happen to you. Having a bloke ferret around trying to find the condom that slipped off is certainly one way to add an element of intimacy to the proceedings, but it's not worth the worry. Get wise, get protection: you'll feel better knowing you're having safe sex and be able to enjoy the rest of it a whole lot more.

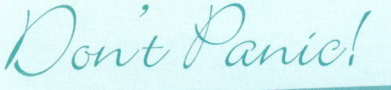

Don't Panic!

THE CONDOM BROKE ...HERE'S WHAT TO DO

- Withdraw immediately.
- Don't douche. Health experts say it can increase your risk of getting an STI from semen or discharge.
- If condoms are your only form of contraception, you can then take emergency contraception to prevent pregnancy. The emergency contraceptive (EC) pill or "the morning after pill" comes in a pack of two pills, each containing the hormone levonorgestrel. The first pill must be taken within three days (72 hours) of having unprotected sex, and the second pill, exactly 12 hours after. If taken this way, EC is about 85 per cent effective in preventing pregnancy. It's available from pharmacists without a prescription.
  - See your GP as soon as possible so you can be checked for STIs. If you have caught something, early treatment may minimise symptoms and clear it up more quickly.

CHAPTER EIGHT

How to put a condom on with your mouth

He'll never say no to this lightening-fast manoeuvre. Take some tips from sexpert Lou Paget who explains her "Italian Method".

Lube your lips with a clear, water-based lubricant. Also place a dollop of lubricant in to the nipple of the condom. Pucker your lips and place the nipple of the condom in your mouth, lubricated side towards him. The rolled up condom is outside your mouth.

Holding the shaft of his penis with one hand, allow the condom to rest on the head and push any air bubbles out of the nipple of the condom with your tongue.

In this position, place your teeth over your lips and push gently and firmly on the rim of the condom to unroll it down the shaft.

If you're not able to push the condom all the way down with your lips, don't worry. Go down as far as you can and finish the job with your hand in the shape of an 'okay' sign.

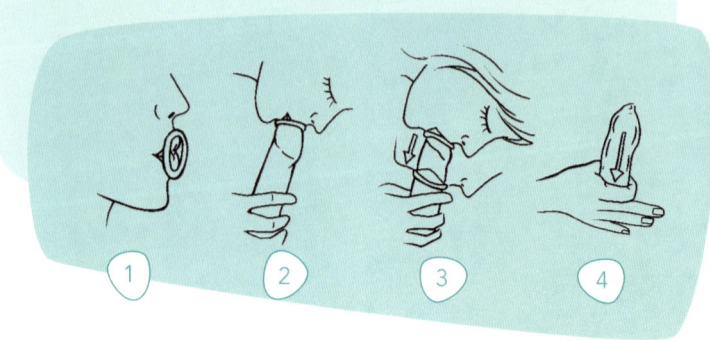

PROTECT YOUR ASSETS

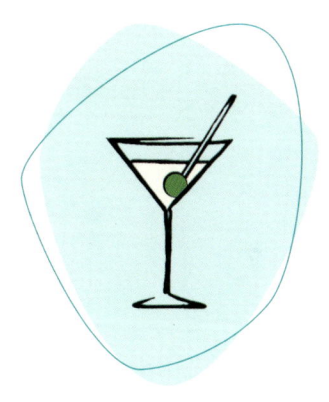

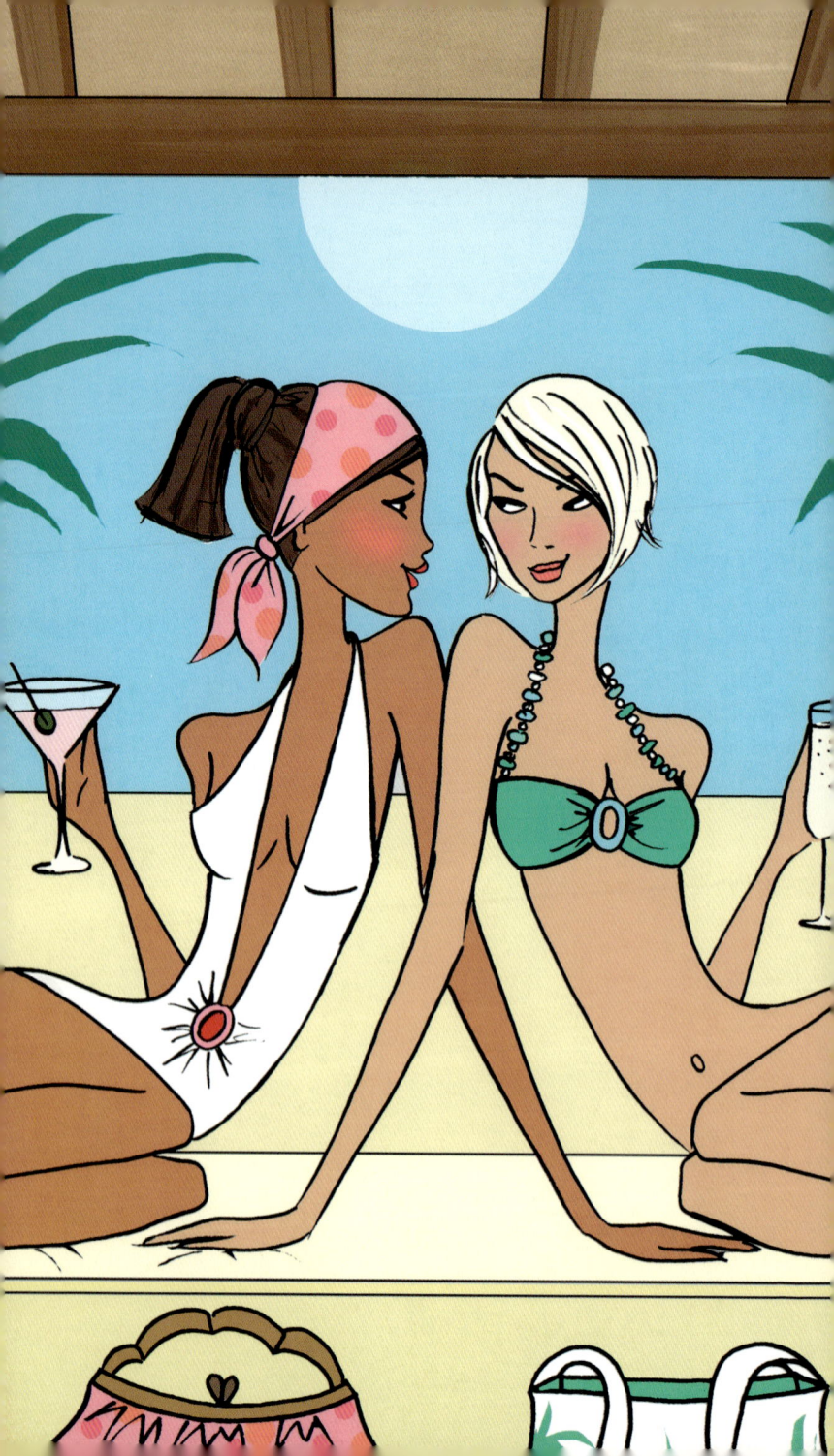

CHAPTER NINE

'Batting For The Other Team'

GAY, LESBIAN, BISEXUAL ...
ARE YOU OR AREN'T YOU?

CHAPTER NINE

I'VE ALWAYS BEEN FASCINATED BY THE IDEA OF BEING WITH ANOTHER WOMAN. OCCASIONALLY, ONE WILL POP UP IN MY FANTASY SHOW REEL. THE OTHER NIGHT, WHILE OUT DANCING, I THINK ONE TRIED TO HIT ON ME. BUT I COULDN'T BE SURE. I'VE NEVER HAD A REAL LESBIAN EXPERIENCE: BAR ONE FUMBLED GROPE WITH A FRIEND WHEN I WAS 13. MUM CALLED US TO COME IN FOR TEA MOMENTS LATER AND THAT WAS THE END OF IT.

It must be fabulous to have someone know instinctively what turns you on and how and where to touch you. In this thought, I am not alone. In the book *Doing It Down Under*, author Juliet Richters says 13 per cent of women have been attracted at least once to someone of the same sex, while 9 per cent have had some form of same-sex sexual experience (against 6 per cent of men).

So whether you've done it, thought about doing it or are just plain curious we thought we'd see how things worked on the other side of the team.

BATTING FOR THE OTHER TEAM

THE GIRL GUIDES

Here it is: everything you want to know about sista-to-sista sex but were hesitant to ask. We put the hard questions to Carol Booth, the author of *Woman To Woman: A Guide To Lesbian Sexuality*.

What do lesbians actually do together?
Lesbian sex often takes longer than hetero sex. Partners are more often aiming for intimacy rather than orgasms, but they're also likely to have greater numbers of multiples than their straight sisters!

What does the foreplay involve?
Many lesbians enjoy talking as a way to ease themselves into sex. Giving or receiving a graphic account of what's about to happen can be very erotic. Just like straight women, many lesbians like the feeling of someone stroking their vulva through their knickers. It's thrilling because it contains a promise of what's to come. Whether it's holding hands, holding her breasts, holding her bum or holding her in your arms, touching is a big turn-on. Kissing is an important part of lovemaking: ears, necks, shoulders, spines, crooks of arms, collarbones, breasts, nipples, navels, ankles, backs of legs, thighs and genitals. Kisses can be feather-light, a little wet with a bit of tongue or very deep. Lesbian sex is no rougher or gentler than heterosexual sex.

Does oral constitute a big part of the sex?
Some of us adore it and others aren't interested. Occasionally, women initially find the smell or taste of another's vagina unappealing, but you and your partner can experiment either by lubricating the area with saliva or by adding flavour

CHAPTER NINE

by way of cream, chocolate, honey or your favourite liqueur.

Do lesbians often penetrate each other?
Once again, some enjoy it, some don't. There's a large market for lesbian-specific dildos and many women enjoy being penetrated by fingers, tongues or even toes.

Do lesbians take masculine (penetrator) and feminine (receiver) roles?
Most lesbian couples would categorise their sexual relationship as being fairly equal and many will penetrate each other, sometimes at the same time. In the past, there tended to be butch/femme role-play, but identifying as butch (more masculine or femme (more feminine) fell out of favour when feminism came along. However, in recent times there has been a resurgence of women interested in exploring the butch/femme dynamic.

What about anal?
Some love it, some enjoy it occasionally and some choose not to do it. Just like straight women.

How do lesbians usually reach orgasm?
Just like straight women: by being fingered, licked, penetrated, kissed and by tribadism, which is rubbing your genitals against the genitals of another person, or another body part, like a leg. Also known as humping. Some can orgasm from having their breasts licked or sucked.

Do lesbians get pissed off when hetero women experiment with gay sex?
Some feel comfortable relating to a woman who may only be exploring. However, there are plenty of stories of lesbians having their hearts broken by straight women who were only

BATTING FOR THE OTHER TEAM

flirting with homosexuality, but then go back to men. So yes, some lesbians feel cautious about straight women.

How do you know if you're lesbian, bisexual or just curious about women?

A lesbian finds her sexual identity over time. However, making love to a woman does not mean you are a lesbian, just as sleeping with a guy doesn't mean that you're straight. Most women sooner or later realise they are either attracted mostly to women, to men or that they are bisexual. There's no need to rush or accept labels. Take time and explore the options available to you.

GIRL-ON-GIRL CONFESSIONS

Lesbian sex. The words would have once brought a flush to your parent's cheeks. Nowadays women are likely to feel a glow somewhere quite different. They look, they linger and they wonder: what would it be like?

"My first sexual experience with a woman was when I had a threesome with her and a man. I discovered I was much more interested in exploring her body than his. So much so, that the next time I saw her, I told her how I felt. I was excited to hear that she fancied me too. That afternoon, we went to her place. I felt something change in me that day: my desires were stronger and the passion was explosive. She traced over every part of my body with her soft tongue while I discovered her inside and out with my hands and mouth. When it arrived, my orgasm was nothing short of earth-shattering and very wet. From that moment on, I knew I was gay and I wouldn't change it for the world."

Tammy, 24.

CHAPTER NINE

"Since I've become a lesbian, I've felt more sexually liberated. The terrain of the female body is completely different and the sex is dynamite. Having sex while wearing a harness is wild. Penetrating my lover in a new way, rather than with my fingers, really turns me on. I love wearing a strap-on – the huge black penis looks amazing and I get to pleasure my girlfriend with it. Putting on wrist and leg restraints, using a riding crop and wearing masks gives us thrills too. The female body is the most beautiful creation in the world and being so close to it feels like a blessing."

Carly, 29.

"One night, Melissa and I went to a rave party and at the end of the evening we caught a taxi home so I could crash at her house. During the night I got up to get a drink and found Melissa's mother Bev in the lounge room watching a porno. At first, I was so shocked I didn't know what to do but then she called me over and asked me to sit down and watch the movie with her. Being a lesbian, it was kind of a turn-on for me because this would be my first experience with an older woman. Then Bev started touching me and I returned the favour. Before I knew it, we were both naked and taking turns to lick each other. There was lots of fondling and it all felt right. Bev was 43 but her body was amazing. The next morning I went home early and Melissa never suspected a thing. To this day, she still has no idea. I sleep over every now and again and Bev and I still fool around."

Wendy 19.

"The great thing about being a lesbian is that it's easier to do it in public without being noticed. You'd be amazed what

BATTING FOR THE OTHER TEAM

you can achieve with a few well-placed hands. My girlfriend and I were at a straight bar last week and we were mingling in a crowd of people. We put our hands down each other's pants and used our fingers to make each other come. It was easy to disguise our 'orgasm faces' under the dimmed lighting but after we did it a second time we realised we should really just go home. No-one had a clue what we'd been up to and that made it all the more exciting."

Emma 25.

"I've tried a double-ended dildo with my lover. It's long and flexible, but takes a fair bit of synchronisation and you need to be quite agile. It feels a bit like you're on a seesaw but it's great because you can go face to face or wrap your legs around each other."

Yvonne 28.

STRAIGHT WOMEN, LESBIAN AFFAIRS

It's a common fantasy. You're happily heterosexual but you've always wondered what it would be like to sleep with a woman. Now, a growing number of straight women are making this fantasy real. What was once taboo has become socially acceptable – even desirable. In fact, it's virtually a sexual trend. But would you do it?

Naomi is a 23-year-old marketing assistant. Two years ago she had a one-night stand with a gay friend.

"I was out to dinner with a friend from work and another friend of hers, Louisa. I'd met Louisa a few times before so I knew she was a lesbian but I'd never given it much thought.

CHAPTER NINE

The three of us went to a Japanese restaurant and drank lots of sake. After dinner we went somewhere else for coffee.

I gradually became aware that Louisa was coming on to me and, oddly enough, it didn't bother me at all. We went on to a club and, soon after we arrived, I said I had to go the bathroom. Louisa followed me and, as we walked down the stairs together, she gently pushed me against the wall and started kissing me. I'd never kissed a girl before and found it a massive turn-on, especially after all that flirting. At that point, I remember thinking two things: 'I hope no-one sees me' and 'I'm about to fulfil one of my sexual fantasies'.

The kissing was totally different to kissing a guy. It just felt so naughty and forbidden. I expected it to be really soft and gentle but she was quite forceful with me. In a funny way, I liked that because, although I was curious, I would never have had the courage to initiate it. When she finally said, 'I'm going home, wanna come?' I said yes straight away before I could change my mind.

We got into the back seat of a cab and kissed all the way to her place. When we got to Louisa's house I could not believe how passionate she was. She threw me down on the couch and kissed me on the mouth, face and neck and unbuttoned my shirt.

Then we went into the bedroom and she slowly undressed me without taking her eyes off my body for a second. I've never experienced a seduction like that; it was just like a scene out of an Anaïs Nin novel. She quickly took her own clothes off and we fell on to the bed.

BATTING FOR THE OTHER TEAM

I'd often fantasised about what it would be like to have another woman give me oral sex and was excited it was about to happen. She pulled me over the edge of the bed and went down on me and I came straight away. But the second after I came, and the sexual tension was released, I felt sick. I thought, 'What am I doing? I have to get out of here.'

The last thing I wanted to do was go down on her and I couldn't bear the thought of lying there in the afterglow. I touched her a bit and we kissed for a little longer but I had this overwhelming desire to get a long way away from the whole situation. I was out the door within 10 minutes of having an orgasm.

Looking back, it was just like when you have a one-night stand with some bastard guy, except I was the guy. I've been in the position where a guy has wanted to leave straight afterwards and I know it doesn't feel fabulous to be left lying there, frustrated, on damp sheets.

Luckily, Louisa had only split from her girlfriend temporarily so she wasn't looking for anything more than a casual fling. We've seen each other quite a few times since that night – at first I felt a bit awkward, but I quickly got over it and we've even joked about our little interlude. I don't think I'd sleep with a woman again. Fantasies are great because you can switch them off at any time, you don't have a living, breathing, horny body beside you to deal with after you come. The nausea I felt after sex with Louisa told me that lesbianism is, for me, better left to my imagination."

CHAPTER NINE

Christina is 26 years old. Although she has had several lesbian affairs, she still considers herself to be heterosexual.

"My boyfriend Simon and I had been together for two years when he first suggested we take home another girl for a threesome. My first reaction was 'No way', but it got me thinking. I'd had gay fantasies before and I certainly enjoyed checking out other women's bodies; I just didn't know whether I could actually go through with it.

After suggesting it the first time, Simon wouldn't give up, insisting it would heat up our sex life. I was still hesitant but I was so in love with him that I was willing to give it a try.

About a month later, we were at a party and an attractive blonde was flirting outrageously with him. At the end of the night Simon introduced me to Miranda and asked if he could bring her home with us for a threesome. I didn't want to disappoint him and I wanted him to see me as a free-thinking, spontaneous person, so I agreed.

When we got back to our flat, Simon went into the kitchen to make coffee and Miranda and I started chatting. We knew a few people in common and shared a similar sense of humour, so by the time Simon joined us we were pretty relaxed.

After a few minutes, Simon just came right out and said, 'So why don't you two kiss?' We both giggled nervously and she began to kiss me.

I couldn't believe how soft her skin was, it was incredible. Simon had a goatee so I was used to a rough texture but Miranda's lips seemed to melt with mine.

BATTING FOR THE OTHER TEAM

While Simon watched, we quickly slipped out of our clothes and began stroking each other all over. She kissed her way down my body until her head was between my legs and then proceeded to give me the best oral sex I'd ever had. I can't remember how many times I came that night. It was just one long series of orgasms and erotic sensations as the three of us had sex for what seemed like hours.

The next day I was surprised at my complete lack of guilt or confusion about sleeping with a woman. The fact that Simon had been part of the experience gave it a kind of heterosexual credibility – like it was just a kinky extension of our normal sex life. Over the next year, we had several more threesomes and I never once considered that I might be gay.

After we broke up, however, I went through a lot of mental anguish about my own sexuality. I couldn't pretend that I hadn't enjoyed sleeping with girls but I'd never done it without Simon being there and taking an active role. If I slept with another woman on my own, would that make me a lesbian?

I knew of a club in the city where there was a girls-only lesbian night on Sundays, so about three months after Simon and I split up, I went there alone with the sole intention of finding a woman to have sex with.

I'd only been at the bar for a couple of minutes when a really cute girl with long, dark hair came up to me and started a conversation. Amy was 26, and after we'd had a few more drinks, she asked me if I wanted to go back to her place.

CHAPTER NINE

Before I knew it we were out the door and in a taxi.

Sex with Amy was definitely different for me. For a start, I didn't feel like I was part of some elaborate sexual performance; it was just the two of us alone in bed together. Perhaps the thought that I might be gay made me too uncomfortable or maybe there wasn't the right chemistry between us – whatever the reason, I just couldn't seem to get into the whole experience with this beautiful girl.

Kissing, caressing and oral sex were fine but it came to the point where I was really hanging out for a penis. Not a cold, plastic dildo or vibrator, but the real thing.

Amy must have sensed something was wrong because she stopped and asked me if I was okay. I reluctantly told her the truth about how confused I was and she was incredibly understanding. I wasn't the first 'straight-experimenting' woman she had slept with and we had a long talk about threesomes and the whole gay-fling thing.

I came to realise that it turned me on to sleep with a woman in the context of a heterosexual relationship – it was a novelty, like anal sex or sex in the shower. And I also get a sexual charge out of having a guy watch me and turning him on as well – maybe it's the exhibitionist in me. Anyway, I found that I find threesomes much more erotic than just me and another woman.

Since that night I've slept with two other women during threesomes. Both times they were part of couples and I was the other woman.

BATTING FOR THE OTHER TEAM

I know I'm not gay. I don't even think I'm bisexual, and I would always be honest about my experiences with future boyfriends. I think it's important to keep an open mind about these things and anyway, it's every guy's fantasy, isn't it?"

Five women you shouldn't pash

- Your boss, colleague or client (unless you're happy to lose your job and/or reputation).
- Your sister-in-law (too close for comfort).
- Your best friend (you risk losing her unless she's in to it-even then tread very, very carefully)
- Someone else's girlfriend (unless all parties know and are happy about it).
- Any girl under the age of consent (carnal knowledge is a criminal offence).

BISEXUAL

This is probably the least understood of sexual choices. Can we be truly inclined to swing both ways or is it just indecision? You decide.

What exactly is bisexuality? That he's deciding whether he's gay? That he touched another boy while he was at school? That he has affairs with men and women at the same time? It's a grey area among the experts. Freud believed bisexuality was a stepping stone to homosexuality. Pioneering sex researcher Dr Alfred Kinsey defined bisexuality as falling

CHAPTER NINE

anywhere between completely heterosexual and completely homosexual. Sex researchers Masters and Johnson identified bisexual men as ranging from a gay man who marries a woman as a cover, to a straight guy who gets an illicit thrill from same-sex relations.

The way to find out whether your man is bisexual may seem obvious: just ask. But the reality is that even if you're courageous enough to risk offending him, the answer you receive could be less than conclusive. Half the men who have had sex with other men do not consider themselves gay or bisexual, according to the largest sex survey in the word (The US National Health and Social Life Survey). So when a man tells you he's straight, it doesn't mean that he hasn't had – and acted on – sexual feelings for another man. Likewise, just because you have a few doubts about his true sexuality, it doesn't mean he's a raving queen.

While a man initiating anal sex may fill a woman's mind with doubts, her fears are probably unfounded. A recent survey by US Playboy magazine found that 47 per cent of 100,000 vehemently heterosexual male readers admitted to having tried anal intercourse with a woman. Dr Jack Morin, a sex therapist and author of a book about anal sex for men and women, believes anal sex is not inherently homosexual. "The anus is an area richly endowed with nerve endings and interconnected with the main pelvic muscles. Yet the powerful taboo surrounding anal eroticism and fear of HIV inhibits many people from experimenting with anal play."

Men typically derive more pleasure from receiving anal penetration than women. In men, the prostate – which is just

BATTING FOR THE OTHER TEAM

beyond the rectal wall – can be a source of pleasure. Also, the lower end of the penis is near the anal opening and is stimulated indirectly by most types of anal sex. "What we're talking about is not an exclusively gay sex act," says Dr Morin. "For most gay, straight or bi men, this is a pleasurable thing. Anal sex can be a healthy part of a normal heterosexual sex life, provided you practice safe sex."

The five things that don't necessarily mean he's bisexual

1. An interest in anal sex.
2 Having gay friends.
3. An interest in fashion, shopping, ballet or show tunes.
4. A dislike of sports and traditional "guy" things.
5. Spending evenings alone.

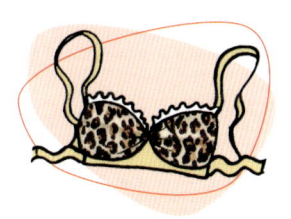

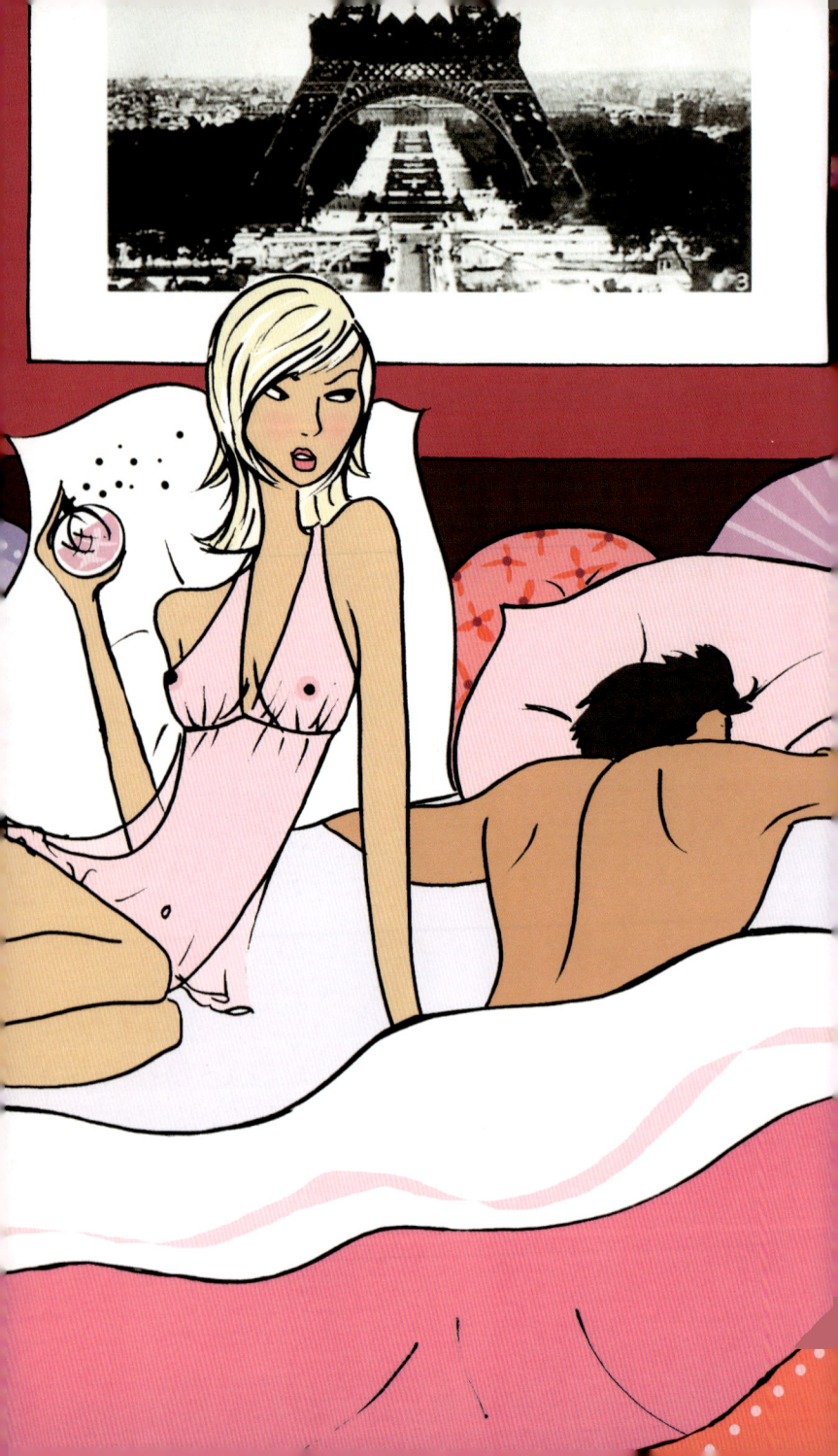

CHAPTER TEN

When good sex goes bad

WHAT CAN GO WRONG?
THE DOS AND DON'TS OF SEX

CHAPTER TEN

I ONCE RUINED A FRIEND'S SHEETS WITH AN OVER ENTHUSIASTIC AMOUNT OF MANGO BODY BUTTER. AT THE TIME IT WAS FANTASTIC, I FELT LIKE I WAS HAVING SEX IN THE TROPICS INSTEAD OF IN MY FRIEND'S RATHER DINGY SPARE ROOM. BUT THE SAID SHEETS WERE RUINED AND IT PROVED TO BE A COSTLY EXPERIENCE (A QUEEN-SIZE SHEET SET OF THE FINEST THREAD COUNT IS NEARLY AS EXPENSIVE AS TEN DAYS IN THE TROPICS, IN FACT).

I have made far worse errors of judgement in the sack than that. I've slept with men I shouldn't have (ones who never called or the type that thank you after sex like you've done them a huge favour). I've put fingers where they weren't welcome, pulled when I should have tugged, and squeezed when I should have stroked. I have made noises that I wished I hadn't made and been relieved that I was facing the other way, lest he witnessed my horrified blushes. When there are so many options and so much at stake it is only natural that a few errors are made along the way.

When it comes to bad sex there is bad, really bad and downright awful. Sometimes it's something silly or

WHEN GOOD SEX GOES BAD

embarrassing. Other times it is something painful. And occasionally it is something unacceptable. It is important to differentiate between the three. Most of the time staying relaxed and in good humour can smooth the occasional bumpy ride. Sometimes serous intervention is needed. So whatever your particular problem may be, we look at what can be done to remedy this situation and bring the raunch factor back in to play.

SEX BLOOPERS

Farts? Weird talk? Small willy? Oh stop, it's easily fixed.

Sometimes things just don't go according to plan. You know what we're talking about. It's those sexual worst case scenarios when your dignity is left hanging tenuously by a thread. We may not be able to stop them happening, but we can help you emerge with your self-esteem in tact.

You got drunk and disgraced yourself

There is nothing wrong with having a few libido loosening wines but polishing off a few bottles is not to be advised. "I went home with this girl once who just seemed a bit tipsy", says Craig, 26. "We started fooling around, and everything was great, until she leant over the couch and vomited on the carpet. It was not a good look."

Survival plan: You might want to start by not downing an entire bottle of champagne before the entrees have arrived. However if you're way past the point of no return and have already shown off your seductive dance moves to the entire restaurant, then it's all about damage control. "The next day, send him a text message or email apologising for your behaviour," suggests Kathy Buchanan, author of Charm

CHAPTER TEN

School: A Girl's Complete Etiquette Handbook. "You may like to say something light-hearted like, 'Sorry, I don't normally get so drunk. I do remember having fun before I passed out. Perhaps you'll give me a chance to redeem myself?'" Then if you get one, try and stay sober.

You tell him "I love you." He says nothing.

Picture this: In the middle of mind-blowing sex with a very cute boy you blurt out those three little words. His reaction? He not only goes cold, he goes limp, literally. Ouch! This is never going to be a good situation but stay calm, turning in to a screaming psycho isn't going to make him fall in love with you any faster.

Survival plan: If you don't get the hoped for response, don't push the issue. You might explain, "I just wanted you to know how I felt". Then change the subject. If you do wish to discuss it further then raise the issue later, out of the bedroom. Casually ask, "Where do you think our relationship is heading?" Hopefully he won't respond: "Out the door, as fast as my legs will carry me."

His weapon is really weenie.

You were expecting a hummer and instead you got a bummer. If his initial unveiling is a let down try to avoid screaming, "What do you call that" or asking "Is it in yet?"

Survival plan: Try to experiment with different positions. In her book Sex In The City, a guide to dating and sex for modern women, Lisa Sussman suggests lying flat on your back with your legs tucked up against your chest. Scrunching up this way will shorten your vagina and create a tighter squeeze. Move around, vary speeds and tell him what feels

WHEN GOOD SEX GOES BAD

good. Failing that, just be thankful he doesn't have a really hairy back.

He's really bad in bed.
First time in the sack should not be held as a benchmark for all that follows. Nerves may be to blame for the fumbling when he should be fondling. If he doesn't make any progress in the sessions that follow then it's worth trying to teach him a few new moves (well, someone has to get him started…)

Survival plan: "Getting what you want in bed is not hard," say Dan Anderson, co-author of Sex Tips For Straight Women From A Gay Man. "Take control and show, or tell, him what you like. Most men will love the fact you want great sex." Try these cringe-free techniques: Say, "I love it when I'm on top." Then just do it. Or, "It makes me so hot when you put your hand right here." Then move it.
Whisper, "Want to know how to really make me wild?" Then show him.

He, um, sorta 'accidentally' sticks it in the wrong hole.
There is no such thing as accidentally. If he heads in that direction it's because that's his intended destination.
Unless he's totally in the dark then, anatomically speaking, he can tell one hole from the other. There's no "Whoops, my mistake" about it.

Survival plan: Yes, most guys are obsessed with back-door sex. If it's not your thing (and you wouldn't be alone), let him know nicely but firmly. Use your hand to guide him back to the right place and then moan pleasurably. He'll get the message.

CHAPTER TEN

Your dirty talk freaks him out.

I've been there - just innocently trying to add a bit of filth to the proceedings, when he looks more alarmed than aroused. Most men like a bit of encouragement every now and again, especially vocal exclamations on his performance ("You feel so hard/big/long/deep") But baby talk, name-calling or nagging are best left well enough alone.

Survival plan: Before you whip out the dirty vocab try and suss if he'll be in to it or not. Completely silent foreplay may indicate he's not much of a talker during sex. But if he's moaning and groaning a bit you can test the waters with a little "Ooh baby, that feels good" and gauge his reaction. If you have already launched in to your full "I'm a dirty little girl" spiel and he's looking at you in horror then stop; laugh it off and tell him you were just fooling around. No point asking, "What's wrong? My ex used to like it." Cause that's just going to hurt.

You let one rip mid-act.

This is not really our fault. They seem to sneak up on you without warning and we are talking from both ends - farting and varting. It happens but why? Well, that's actually due to excess air being pushed in each time he thrusts. So they are perfectly normal, usually odourless but nonetheless painfully blush-making.

Survival plan: Relax. Men are not as stressed about bodily functions as we women are (take note of how freely they fart, burp, snore). Usually they are far more concerned with the sex to let the odd fanny fart stop them mid-stride. If it's a one-off, best to ignore it. If it's closer to World War III, a simple "Oops, sorry" is all you really need.

WHEN GOOD SEX GOES BAD

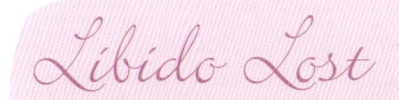

Libido Lost

You used to rip each other's clothes off, now you'd rather watch the telly. Wondering where your libido has gone and how you can get it back? Some lifestyle choices have a direct impact on your sexual performance. Guilty as charged?

BOOZE: Excessive consumption can cause impotence for him ("brewers droop"), a lack of sensation for you and, in severe cases, impotence.

SLOTH: If you're a couch potato, is it any surprise you're not a horn-bag? Sex requires a degree of fitness, so healthy lungs, stamina and being in your correct weight range will help.

CIGGIES: Don't be fooled by the post-coital puff enjoyed in the movies. Welcome to real life, where smoking is about bad breath, clogged arteries and in extreme cases, an impairment of sperm production - not much of a mood maker.

HE CAN'T GET IT UP. IS IT YOUR FAULT?

Let us pity the poor penis for a moment (not an emotion usually associated with this forthright member). By day, he goes about his no-frills job of flushing fluid from the body. Then, especially as an apprentice, there's the seemingly gazillion unscheduled, unwanted and sometimes inexplicable erections. Tired and yawning? Erection. See a pretty girl? Erection. Riding a bike and the penis falls between your inner

CHAPTER TEN

thighs as you pedal? Erection. Then there's the morning glory when the bed looks like a marquee with the penis acting as tent pole. This one is less likely to be about your splendid beauty in the morning and a lot more to do with him trying to hold in a wee big enough to douse a bushfire.

Despite this exhausting and relentless schedule-over which men have very little control incidentally-he is then supposed to transform in to some sort of military Don Juan at night. Standing to attention, on-call to satisfy his partner (as well as himself) at the drop of a hat. Or pants. That's a lot of pressure for a 12cm muscle... it's a demanding life and sometimes the strain shows in poor performance. Or non-performance. There are a few reasons why your boyfriend can't get it up, and hardly any of them are your (or his) fault.

The Obvious: If you are getting hot and heavy - especially with a younger guy - the likely reason he can't get it up is because he's already blown his load. In all the excitement he may have ejaculated prematurely or Ben-Stiller style, he may have jerked off earlier to ensure going the distance. Either way he will be keeping quiet. Best just to try again later.

Not in the mood: Despite common perceptions guys aren't always in the mood to have sex. Sometimes they are just too tired, stressed, too whatever to get it up. A girl can go ahead anyway and fake it if need be (not that I am condoning that) but a man can't fake an erection. Nothing that a good night's sleep or a comforting chat can't heal. Nothing to stress about.

Performance anxiety: The shy cousin of drunkenness, but probably not quite as common, is the male fear of not being

WHEN GOOD SEX GOES BAD

good enough. This is particularly likely if the woman is intimidating or he considers her out of his league. Stage fright can result in nothing happening, which is only marginally better than prematurely ejaculating. I'd take this one as a compliment and do my best to soften the blow.

Ups and Downs: In a new relationship desire to have sex is far stronger than when things become more established. Once a few months pass and a couple finds a pattern and routine, the erotic dust inevitably settles. When you know you can probably get it tomorrow night, that burning sense of must-have-you-now lust fades. So occasionally, he decides to hibernate. If this is happening regularly, it's time to spice things up. Don't read too much in to it - welcome to the peaks and troughs of normal life.

None of the above: Once you've eliminated the above reasons, it's time to worry. He's either got a medical condition or the relationship is in trouble. It could mean he's not attracted to you anymore. It could also signal he's having an affair and getting his fix elsewhere. These things need to be discussed. If it is about your relationship, counselling is a highly effective route; if it's medical, a doctor is the only route. Although it's hard to persuade the average male to seek help - especially when it comes to discussing his penis and the word flaccid in the same sentence. Peer pressure dictates that if there's one thing a man should be able to do, it's getting it up. If they can't accomplish that, what can they do? So, if you want to broach the subject, tread carefully.

CHAPTER TEN

Mr Floppy :: The Medical Facts

Okay, enough of the jokes already. Erectile dysfunction (ED) is a medical condition described as "the inability for a man to achieve and maintain an erection sufficient for satisfactory sexual activity." Research by Impotence Australia indicates that around a third of Australian men will experience ED at some point, yet only 11 per cent will consult a doctor.

According to Sydney based GP Dr Denise Lerino, "ED is a very common medical condition and one that, we need to emphasise to men and their partners, is treatable like any other."

ED can be caused by a host of factors such as:
• Diabetes, hypertension or heart disease. • Spinal or pelvic injuries. • Treatments such as radiotherapy or anti depressant medication. • Psychological factors such as depression, bereavement or fatigue.

These may sound like things that only apply to older people but there are other contributing factors young people are particularly disposed to; alcohol, recreational drugs and smoking.

There are a range of treatments for ED ranging from counselling, exercises, penile implants and pumps, to injections and Viagra (which works by relaxing the blood vessels in the penis during sexual excitement, allowing blood to flow to the area and an erection to occur in the natural way.)

So, there is no need for embarrassment and everything to gain by getting it "fixed" and back in firing form.

WHEN GOOD SEX GOES BAD

WHEN SEX HURTS:
Why it hurts and what you can do about it.

Most of us are only too aware that love hurts. There's no pain quite as excruciating as feeling your heart breaking. Sex, on the other hand, should never be painful though at some point you may find it is. The cause may be a serious infection but more commonly, it's the result of an easily treated infection or allergy. Or it could be due to stress, anxiety or over-enthusiasm. Whatever the cause, pain during sex should always be checked out by your GP. Persevering when your body just doesn't feel right (in the hope you'll get going) is definitely not the answer, and the one thing that you can be sure will suffer is your sex life. It's too easy to get caught in a vicious circle where previous pain or discomfort makes you anxious the next time you have sex - and that anxiety makes sex even more painful!

Pain on Entry

Dry vagina: Probably the most common cause of superficial pain. This can be due to your partner's over-eagerness to get down to business. When a woman becomes sexually aroused, the walls of her vagina secrete a fluid that makes it moist and ready for her partner's penis. How long you need to get turned on depends on your mood, the time of the month and how sexy you feel. Our bodies don't work like clockwork. Where you are in your menstrual cycle can make your vagina drier than normal. Women who are breastfeeding often find they need additional lubrication. Stress in your daily life or 'first night' nerves with a new man can also be factors.

Treatment: It's been said before, but it's worth saying again

CHAPTER TEN

(and giving your partner timely reminders) that the more time you spend on foreplay, the better sex will feel in the end. But the odd not-so-great night should be kept in proportion. The occasional off night doesn't mean your sex life is doomed - just take more time to get relaxed, wind down and try a long, hot soak. Corny, but it does work.

Oral Contraception: Some women swear that the pill can cause vaginal dryness although doctors disagree. Certainly, higher levels of progesterone do make things a bit drier.

Treatment: There are more 30 brands of oral contraception, so changing brands can solve the problem. You should allow three months for your body to adjust to the changes so don't get in to a swapping frenzy till your body has had time to adapt.

Vaginismus: Some women have deeply unconscious fears or anxieties about penetrative sex that the muscles in the lower third of their vagina go in to spasms - this is known as vaginismus. It can make sex very uncomfortable or even impossible. The muscle spasm is completely involuntary and often women with this condition feel as horny and frustrated as their partner does.

Treatment: Psychosexual counsellors have experience in this area and can help you break the cycle of pain, anxiety and more pain. Alternatively you can contact the sexual health clinic in your area. Check the Yellow Pages for details.

Thrush: Candida albicans is the bane of many women's lives. Yeast that lives happily in the vagina, at times can be triggered into over-production. It is also known as Thrush and causes a hot, burning sensation around the vaginal entrance and the vulva, as well as a thick white discharge that looks like cottage cheese. Thrush makes the skin dry and if you have intercourse you may feel very tender afterwards. Sex when not properly lubricated can also trigger an attack of thrush.

Treatment: A combined prescribed course of cream and pessaries (possibly taken by your partner too). Many women find a tampon dipped in natural yoghurt is equally as effective.

Cystitis: Cystitis is a very painful inflammation of the bladder that causes a burning pain when you urinate, as the acidic urine hits inflamed and sensitive skin. Most women suffer from it at some time or another and unfortunately sufferers tend to get it more than once. Often the treatment for cystitis will trigger Thrush (it's a cruel, cruel world). Cystitis can be caused by infection or bruising of the bladder tissue often through over enthusiastic sex or sex with not enough lubrication. Also making love when your bladder or bowels are full can trigger an attack.

Treatment: As soon as you feel cystitis coming on, drink as much water as you can and wash your bottom gently from front to back every time you go to the toilet. Symptoms can be lessened by drinking special anti-acid cystic drinks (such as Ural and Citravescent) from the chemist. Always consult your doctor if the symptoms continue more than a couple of days, as infection can spread to your kidneys. As a preventative measure, drinking Cranberry juice can be of help.

Allergic reactions: Spermicidal creams can cause allergic reactions, leading to intense itching and swelling around the

CHAPTER TEN

vulva. Using anything highly perfumed around your vagina, such as bubble baths, soaps, sprays or douches, can irritate the skin badly, especially if there any tiny abrasions there to start with.

Treatment: If you suspect spermicides are the problem, try a different brand or condoms without spermicide. For cleansing, stick to unperfumed, pure soaps or plain, warm water. Douching is not a good idea. Your vagina is naturally moist and secretes all the fluids needed to keep it healthy; douching throws the balance out and can lower your resistance to infection and cause dryness.

Deep Pain Inside

Sometimes deep thrusting during sexual intercourse can cause pain right inside your body. This can be a warning sign of infections, which although serious can be treated.

Pelvic Inflammatory Disease (PID): This can be a serious threat to women's fertility, because if left untreated, it will "glue" your reproductive organs together and make you sterile. About 13 in every 1,000 women in Australia are estimated to carry PID. And because the disease can appear to "clear up" and be completely without symptoms, doctors estimate many women are unaware they have the infection.

Pelvic Inflammatory disease is an umbrella term for infections or inflammations that have penetrated deep in to the reproductive system - it can hit the ovaries, fallopian tubes and/or the uterus. It can be caused by a number of means, but often it is caused by Chlamydia or gonorrhoea contracted through sexual intercourse with an infected partner, which then spreads to their tubes. Left untreated, PID not only affects fertility, it can also lead to chronic ill health. In the early stages, pain can be so mild you may not notice it or maybe just feel an ache in the abdomen during or after intercourse.

Treatment: PID is treatable but the earlier it is caught, the less damage is likely to occur. Early diagnosis is treated with antibiotics, bed rest and abstinence. If it's serious a hospital stay may be necessary. In extreme cases surgery may be required. If PID is suspected, your doctor should always do a test for gonorrhoea and Chlamydia. Without sounding alarmist it is well worth visiting a sexual health clinic every time you change sexual partners as some sexually transmitted diseases, such as Chlamydia, can be symptom-free.

Endometriosis: Every month, the cells that make up the lining of the womb are released as a period if no fertilised egg arrives. Endometriosis occurs when the cells of this tissue travel outside the uterus and begin growing elsewhere in the body. The growths are usually found in the pelvic area but have been found as far away as inside the nose. The pain will depend on where the growth is - a growth on one of the uterine ligaments can get bumped deep inside during intercourse, which is very painful indeed.

Treatment: This depends on the amount of endometrial patches there are. You can have them removed surgically or by laser treatment, or use drugs to shrink the cysts and minimise the pain.

Ectopic Pregnancy: In rare cases an ectopic pregnancy, when the egg is lodged and growing in the fallopian tube

CHAPTER TEN

can cause dull pain during intercourse. It is not a common symptom-usually women experience mild bleeding, abdominal tenderness and missed or abnormal periods. Many women experience all the normal signs of pregnancy such as nausea and swelling of the breasts.

Treatment: If diagnosed early, surgery will be required to remove the embryo. If undiagnosed the embryo can rupture the fallopian tube requiring urgent surgery.

Cysts: Sometimes ovaries develop harmless cysts. These are common and often don't cause any symptoms or discomfort. Most cysts are fluid filled sacs that develop on one or both of your ovaries. They can cause pain during sex, a swollen stomach or upset your monthly cycle. They usually disappear by themselves but may grow to an extent they put pressure on surrounding organs. Occasionally they need to be treated either with surgery or hormone therapy.

Contraceptive discomfort: Diaphragms come in different shapes and sizes and badly-fitting diaphragms can be uncomfortable. You should have your diaphragm checked every seven months to check it is the correct size for you as weight changes, childbirth or pregnancy terminations can alter the size you need. Although intra-uterine devices (IUD's) which go inside your uterus, have had bed press in the past, they are now considered perfectly safe. However, if you use an IUD and feel pain during sex, you should have it checked out by your GP.

Deep pain during sex needn't always be a sign of such serious problems but it is always worth consulting your GP to discover its cause.

WHEN GOOD SEX GOES BAD

Remember: love might hurt but sex shouldn't.

HIGH PRESSURE SEX

In these sexually-liberal times (where we know what turns us on and carry condoms just in case) it is surprising how many of us still have trouble saying no to sex we don't really want. Why do we still wake up next to someone and feel uncomfortable and ashamed? The answer is usually because we feel under some sort of pressure. After a few drinks, you might hook up with some man and by the time you realise you aren't too keen things have already heated up. And instead of excusing yourself from the situation you have sex with him. It's easier than arguing or have him thinking you led him on. Or you agree to something that you feel very uncomfortable doing to save being labelled a prude.

If you've ever had sex in these less than ideal circumstances you're not the only one. A recent survey found that nearly 50 per cent of young women engaged in sex with someone they didn't really want to. When asked why 30 per cent said they felt under pressure from the man, 26 per cent felt they'd led him on (turning the blame inwards is very common) and 20 per cent were too embarrassed to say no. The remaining 39 per cent said they went ahead with sex because it was easier than arguing. Many smart, independent women, who can forcefully assert their opinion in a meeting or argue a point in the courtroom, have found themselves relinquishing power in the bedroom.

High-pressure sex shouldn't be confused with date rape, although the line between them is blurry; the difference lies in the use of force. Date rape often involves a degree

CHAPTER TEN

of physical force, but may also be marked by intense intimidation or other forms of psychological coercion, like social or emotional blackmail. Another crucial point is the woman clearly expresses her lack of consent in an obvious way; either verbally by saying "No" or "I don't want to" or by expressing emotional distress or anger - and the date rapist ignores or pretends to misread her.

Unlike date rape, which isn't consensual at all, high-pressure sex is ambiguous because it does involve some form of consent. It relies more heavily on manipulation and subtler forms of psychological warfare: pleading, presuming or wearing the other person down. While the date rapist exploits a woman's terror, the man in a high-pressure sex scenario plays on emotions like pity, guilt, insecurity and embarrassment.

So, why is "No" such a difficult word to say? On paper, some of our reasons for agreeing to sex we don't want seem trite. We might not want to be seen as a bad date, or to be labelled a "tease" or a "prude". We may need to feel that men find us attractive. In a lot of cases we do actually want to have sex with them at some point in the future, but not right this minute. It's hard to draw the line and ask for what we really do want. A little breast fondling and a kiss goodnight? Oral sex but no intercourse tonight thank you? Our culture teaches us not to talk about these things and so we end up doing things we don't want to.

Men aren't always the villains
What makes high-pressure sex even harder to deal with is that in some cases no-one is to blame. The guy - far from

WHEN GOOD SEX GOES BAD

being an assailant - is baffled about what his partner wants, and honestly believes she wants to have sex. Many women assume that men can interpret their body language and read the subtle signals that say she doesn't want to go further. But there are also the men who don't try to understand. They are the ones who've bought into an idea that still permeates popular culture: women secretly long to be sexually dominated. These men rely on the implied passive threat of physical violence to get their way, and women end up having sex that stems from fear.

Women bully their boyfriends too

Women aren't the only ones feeling pressured. 16 per cent of men in a recent survey said they'd been blackmailed, guilt-tripped or otherwise psychologically coerced into intercourse, says Cindy Struckman-Johnson, an expert in sexually aggressive women. While male and female "bullies" have some similarities - there is a distinct difference in how victims from each gender cope. "Women who've been sexually intimidated tend to avoid sex and men in general," says Struckman-Johnson, while men who say they have been "strongly affected" by a traumatic incident try to steer clear of particularly aggressive women, but still retain the same openness toward women and relationships.

CHAPTER TEN

How to make sure it won't happen to you.

Women need to realise they are fully entitled to say no, at any stage of the proceedings. They should practice saying it out loud. "Come up with five sentences you can say to a date, like 'I don't want to do this' or 'I have to go because I need to get up early for work'," advises Madeline Breckinridge, a social worker. If you've had high-pressure sex in the past you need to work out why. It might be that you have a fear of rejection or are worried about disappointing yourself. Understanding why you cave in to the pressure is the first step to unlearning that behaviour and making positive changes. Realise every time you "give in" you're chipping away at your belief and your right and power to speak up. Finally we need to take these experiences seriously. Because as long as we keep quiet about high-pressure sex and its consequences, it will go unrecognised.

> **Remember:** Non-consensual sex (as opposed to high-pressure sex) is rape and is totally unacceptable in all circumstances. If you need help log onto: www.nswrapecrisis.com.au or call your local Rape Crisis Center.

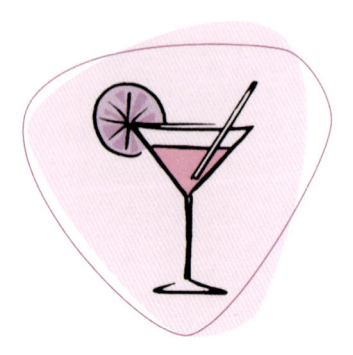

WHEN GOOD SEX GOES BAD

"My most cringe-worthy sex moment"

"I went to a friend's house with a few mates to kick on after a night out. One of the guys suggested we crash in one of the bedrooms. When it became obvious we both wanted to have sex, we looked for lube. There wasn't any in the house, so we decided to use cooking oil. But I had an allergic reaction to the oil and came out in blisters. He had to take me to the hospital and everyone had a laugh at my expense."

Katelyn, 22

"I'd been seeing this guy for a few weeks before he invited me back to his place. I was surprised when we arrived at his parent's house and he asked me to sneak in the back door. What really freaked me out was when I saw he had a single bed - with a racing car cover and mobile airplanes hanging from the ceiling. I decided to bail."

Vicki, 27

"I suffer from bad asthma and if I have an attack it can be life-threatening. I met this sexy, sophisticated guy and we were getting passionate at my place. Suddenly I heard this wheezing grunt. It kept getting louder until I realised he was heaving as loudly as a tractor. Before I knew it, on came the light and my dad was standing at the bedroom door in his Y-fronts, holding my puffer."

Madeline, 21.

I'LL HAVE WHAT SHE'S HAVING

BIBLIOGRAPHY

'Urge' by Dr. Gabrielle Morrissey

'Loving Sex' by Nitya Lacroix

'The Joy of Sex' by Alex Comfort

"Super Sex" by Tracey Cox

"Tantric Sex For Women" by Christina Schulte

"203 Ways To Drive A Man Wild In Bed" by Olivia St Claire

"Women's Pleasure Or How To Have An Orgasm….As Often As You Want" by Rachel Swift

"Mouth Music Made Easy" by Henry Youngberry

"Sex Tips" by Jo-Anne Baker

"The Art Of Sensual Loving" by Anne Hooper

"How To Stay Lovers For Life" by Sharon Wolf

"Well Rounded-Eight Simple Steps For Changing Your Life…Not Your Size" by Catherine Lippincott

"50 Ways To Please Your Lover While You Please Yourself" by Dr. Lonnie Barbach

"The Dance Of Anger" Dr. Harriet Lerner

"Woman To Woman: A Guide To Lesbian Sexuality" by Carol Booth

"365 Days of Sensational Sex" by Lou Paget

"Secrets of the Superyoung" by Dr David Week

"Sexopedia" by Anne Hooper

"A Woman's Complete Guide to Sex" by Susan Quilliam

"The Art of Female Ejaculation" by Lisa S Lawless

"Doing it Down Under" by Juliet Richards and Chris Rissel

"Charm School: A Girl's Complete Etiquette Handbook"

"Sex in the City" by Lisa Sussman

"Sex Tips for Straight Women From a Gay Man" by co-author Dan Anderson

"Unruly Appetites: Erotic Stories" by Hanne Blank

"Naked Erotica" edited by Alison Taylor

"Sweet Life: Erotic Fantasies for Couples" by Violet Blue

CONTACT LIST

CONTACT LIST

Classes and Workshops

Dianne Irvine Orgasm workshop - Coordinator
of sexual concerns and relationships. (08) 8376 6611

Bobbis Pole Studio: (0425) 276 951
(Sydney lap/pole/exotic dance classes)

Showgirls Bar: (03) 9629 4684 (Melbourne pole dancing classes)

Men's Gallery (Melbourne pole dancing classes)

Helplines

Bi-Curious - Need to talk?
Acon from 11am - 12noon or 3 - 5pm on
freecall 1800 063 060 (for one on one counselling)

ACT: Wish - (02) 6257 4915 (6 - 10pm Tuesdays)

NSW: Gay & Lesbian Counselling Service - (02) 8594 9596
or 1800 184 527 (5.30pm - 10.30pm, 7 days)

QLD: Lesbianline - (07) 3252 2997 (7pm - 10pm, 7 days)

SA: Gay & Lesbian Counselling Service - (08) 8334 1623
(7pm - 10pm weekdays, 2pm - 5pm weekends)

TAS: Gayline Tasmania - (03) 6234 8179

VIC: Gay & Lesbian Switchboard - (03) 9827 8544
(6pm - 10pm, 7days)

WA: Gay & Lesbian Community Services
(08) 9420 7201 (7pm - 10pm Mon-Fri)

NT: Consider calling SA or WA helplines.

Websites

www.adultshop.com.au
www.tantra.com
www.holisticwisdom.com
www.fpahealth.org.au
www.pleasurespot.com.au
www.bodyartdoctor.com
www.forthegirls.com
www.sssh.com
www.ninemsn.com.au/cleo
www.cleansheets.com
www.clitical.com
www.thefacts.com.au
www.asexuality.org
www.nswrapecrisis.com.au
www.safepiercing.org
www.couplespleasuredome.com
www.polestars.com.au

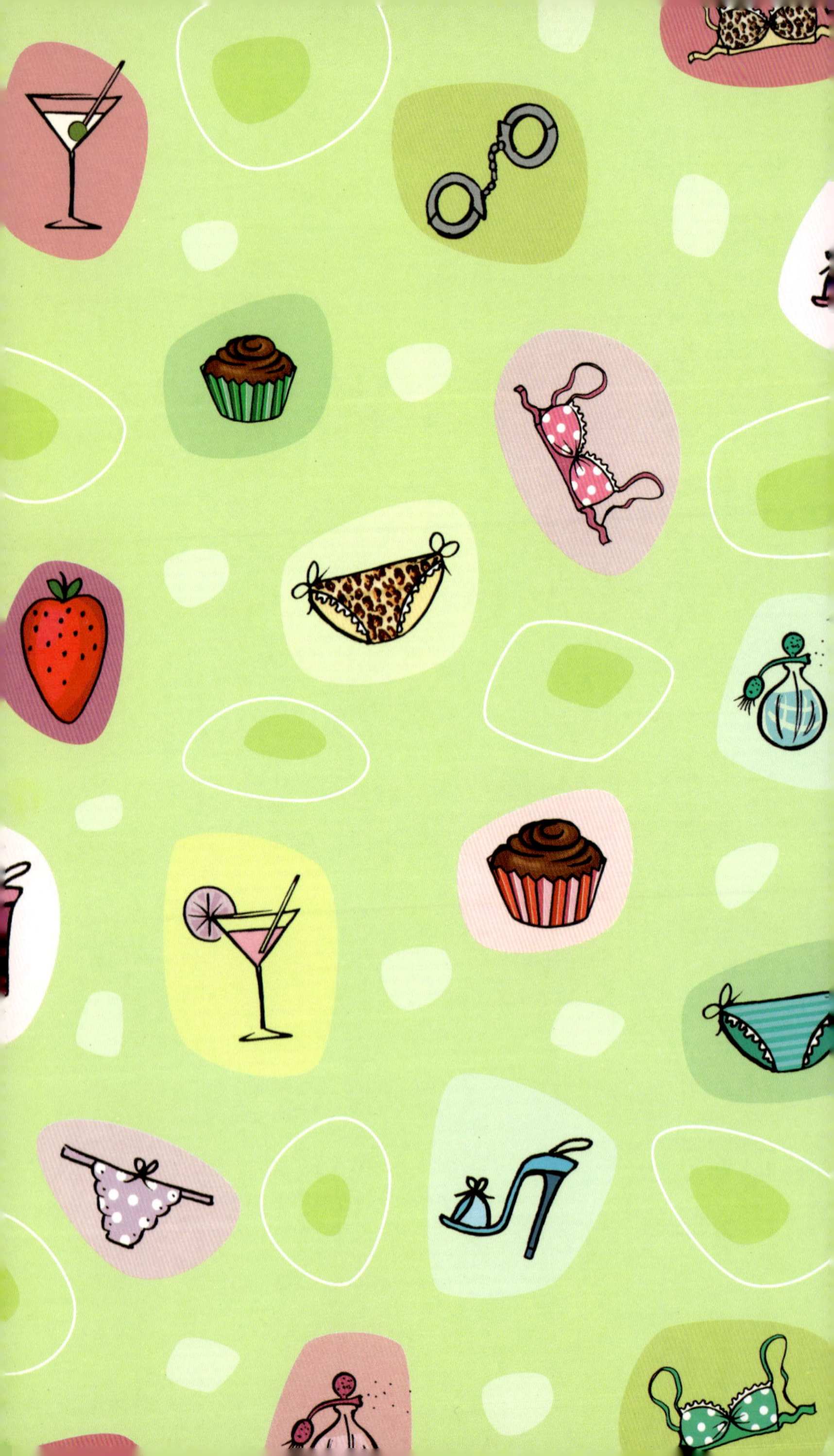